yin
yoga

yin yoga

stretch the mindful way

Kassandra Reinhardt

Contents

Yin sequences

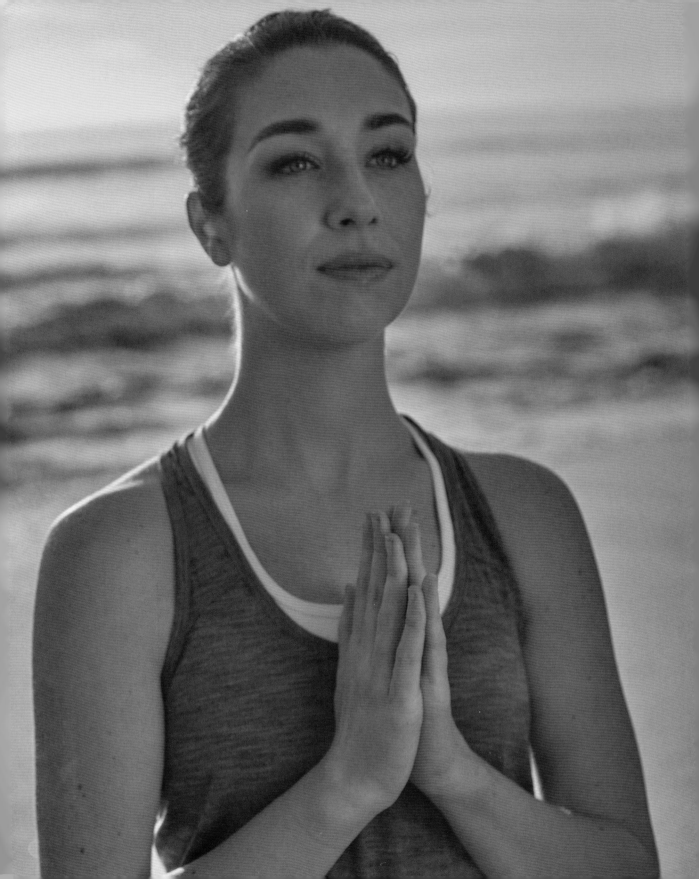

Welcome to yin yoga

Please join me on this journey to learn about this slow-paced style of yoga that can provide a gateway to a way of life filled with more relaxation, greater mindfulness, and less stress. While other yoga forms might push you to strengthen and tone your body, yin yoga invites you to be exactly as you are.

Yin yoga has something to offer to everyone, regardless of your reason for picking up this book and getting on your yoga mat. If you're interested in the physical practice of yoga, you'll enjoy the added flexibility and joint health you feel. But if it's the emotional and mental benefits you seek, you'll find techniques to increase your mindfulness and to decrease your stress.

For years, I only practised stronger styles of yoga, such as vinyasa and power yoga. Although I absolutely loved them, I often found myself feeling physically and emotionally drained. I was regularly stressed, found it hard to fall asleep at night, and couldn't meditate for more than 5 minutes at a time. On a hunch, I tried my first yin yoga class – and it was exactly what I needed!

Most of us lead lives that are already yang in nature, meaning we're active and sometimes even overly active. By only practising yang styles of yoga and leading a busy life, I was burning myself out and not giving myself the chance to slow down and recharge my batteries.

Yin yoga offered me the opportunity to soothe my nervous system, to let go of the need to be always busy, and to learn to truly relax and be in the present moment.

Today, my life and my yoga practice represent a balance between yin and yang. Because of yin yoga, I know how to properly cope with stress, I fall asleep easily, and I genuinely enjoy sitting in meditation. I feel healthier, calmer, and much more flexible – physically and mentally.

This book's intention is to give you the information you need to begin practising yin yoga at home on your own. Of course, receiving guidance from a teacher in person is tremendously beneficial, but doing yoga at home is a great way to be consistent in your practice. It also gives you the freedom to create your own sequences and the power to learn what your body needs at any given moment.

I hope this book brings you the gift of physical, mental, and emotional health. Most of all, I hope it inspires you to take the first step towards creating more balance in your life.

Kassandra Reinhardt

Yin yoga is a practice of *self-love* and *self-acceptance*

About yin yoga

Within this chapter you'll learn yin yoga philosophies, principles, and techniques that can help you prepare your mind, body, and physical space for a safe and mindful yin yoga experience.

What is yin yoga?

When you hear the word "yoga", you might think of such styles as ashtanga, which is physically demanding and requires extreme focus, or bikram (often referred to as "hot yoga"), which is performed in heated rooms and results in a whole lot of sweat. But yin yoga is different.

The practice

In ancient Chinese philosophy, yin and yang describe how seemingly opposite forces are connected and can help bring balance. This belief also applies to the practice of yoga.

A different style Yin and yang yoga styles move energy throughout the body and help improve physical, mental, and emotional wellbeing. But yin yoga offers two components that yang yoga lacks: a focus on stillness and an emphasis on longer, deeper stretching of the tissues that surround your body's moving parts. While most yang styles move quickly and focus on muscle tissues, yin yoga moves slowly and stretches more deeply into the body.

A deeper stretch While most forms of yoga focus on building muscle strength and increasing flexibility, yin yoga centres on stretching deeper connective tissues, such as ligaments, tendons, and deep fascia – the tissue that surrounds muscles. This deeper connection is why yin yoga is often called "yoga of the joints".

A passive practice Because you perform yin yoga while sitting or lying down in a passive manner, gravity plays a role in developing a deeper stretch while enabling you to hold postures for longer periods of time. In yin yoga, instead of contracting your muscles to build strength or elevating your heart rate to build stamina, you're encouraged to relax and surrender to gravity.

The principles

Sarah Powers, a pioneer of yin yoga, defined three universally acknowledged principles for every practice, which together form the basis for practising yin yoga safely and effectively.

Find your edge Finding your edge – knowing when to stop during a posture – helps create the essential balance between no sensation and too much sensation in the body. You can learn your edge by stopping at a point during a posture where you feel intense sensations. If you go beyond that point, you risk injury.

Be still Once you find your edge, you remain still. Paying attention to your tendency to fidget, move, or mentally distract yourself is the purpose of being still. By achieving a meditative state, you're better able to listen to your body and honour your limits. Being still is critical to your yin yoga practice.

Hold the posture You'll gain the most from your yin yoga practice by holding a posture. While beginning practitioners might start with a 1- to 3-minute hold time, more experienced students might hold asanas anywhere from 5 to 10 minutes.

Ancient origins – modern practice

Yin yoga blends teachings from two different lineages: traditional Indian hatha yoga and the Chinese Taoist yin yang philosophy. Each asana – Sanskrit for "manner of sitting" – is derived from hatha yoga, but the process of holding postures for an extended period of time is rooted in Chinese Taoist practices.

Today, yin yoga serves as the antidote to your often busy and stress-filled life, which is typically yang in nature. Too much yang activity can cause an imbalance on physical, emotional, and mental levels. While you never want to be completely yin, true health and wellbeing come from the practice of balancing the yin and the yang, the passive and the active, and the calming and the stimulating.

Why do yin yoga?

Yin yoga targets your physical, mental, and emotional concerns through deep stretching and breathing. However, unlike most yang styles of yoga – which typically focus on stretching muscles and emphasize shorter hold times – yin yoga reaches deeper into your body and mind.

Physical benefits

Your physical body will benefit most from practising yin yoga because it touches every element of your musculoskeletal system. Yin yoga focuses on your fascia – tissue around muscles and organs – so you should feel improved health on the inside, which should improve how you feel on the outside.

Improved joint health The primary physical benefit of yin yoga is strengthening the connective tissues in your joints. They're strengthened through steady, sustained stretching. By applying stress to your joints through stretching, yin yoga helps open and lubricate tight joints.

Increased mobility As you age, you start to lose joint mobility. It's therefore essential to keep your hip, lower back, and pelvic areas healthy and flexible, so you can remain mobile. Yin yoga can free up those areas to increase the range of motion and improve flexibility, making movement and mobility freer and easier.

Better organ function Yin yoga is thought to benefit your heart and lungs through increased blood flow and deeper breathing. Many asanas also include moves that compress and decompress your abdomen, which is believed to help stimulate your digestive system and promote healthier kidney and intestine functions.

Mental and emotional benefits

In addition to physical benefits, like improved digestion, better mobility, and cardiovascular health, practising yin yoga on a regular basis can help to alleviate feelings of stress and anxiety, improve your sleep, and have a positive effect on your mental and emotional states.

Stillness of the mind Yin yoga has a deeply meditative quality that allows you to quieten an overactive mind and tune in to your immediate surroundings. When you remove external stimuli and surrender to the present moment, you can enter a meditative state and let go of mental clutter to achieve a greater sense of inner peace and calm.

Relief from stress Remaining in a high-alert state may contribute to health issues, including high blood pressure and heart problems. Certain asanas could help lower blood pressure and slow down your heart rate to create a greater sense of calm.

Emotional healing When your body is still and your mind is silent, certain feelings – such as sadness, excitement, or anger – can arise during or shortly after practice. Experiencing these emotions is perfectly normal and a healthy effect; your task is simply to observe them as they move through you.

What are chakras?

According to ancient Eastern traditions, *chakras* (Sanskrit for "wheels" or "discs") are energy points within your spiritual body through which *prana* – your life force or life energy – travels.

How chakras work

Yin yoga encompasses more than just postures and breathing exercises for your physical body. It may also have a positive impact on your energetic body by clearing your chakras. It's thought that these energy centres allow for the flow of *prana* through your body, helping to promote physical, mental, and emotional wellbeing.

The tenets of this ancient philosophy say that when your chakras are blocked, you can experience physical maladies, such as muscle tightness or joint stiffness, or emotional manifestations, such as recurring fears or negative emotions. It's believed that practising yin yoga can help clear chakras of energetic blockages and restore their balance.

The seven chakras and their bijas

Repeating aloud a mantra – called a *bija*, which means "seed" in Sanskrit – can unlock each chakra's energy. A *bija* is a sound that should be verbalized and sustained for the length of an exhale. Once the exhale is complete, breathe in and repeat the *bija* for the next exhale.

Chakra	Governs	When balanced	Bijas and asanas
Crown (*sahasrara* in Sanskrit)	Your connection to the universe and is associated with spirituality and enlightenment	You'll feel more connected and more blissful	Bija mantra: OM (or silence) Suggested asanas: any breathing technique, Seated meditation, or Corpse
Third eye (*ajna* in Sanskrit)	Your mind and inner wisdom and is associated with insight, psychic awareness, and imagination	You'll feel better able to tap into your intuition more deeply and see the bigger picture more easily	Bija mantra: OM Suggested asana: Child's pose
Throat (*vishuddha* in Sanskrit)	Your ability to communicate with others and speak the truth and is associated with self-expression, discernment, and honesty	You'll feel more free to speak what's on your mind and in your heart while also learning to be a better listener	Bija mantra: HAM Suggested asana: Neck release
Heart (*anahata* in Sanskrit)	Your ability to relate and empathize with others and is associated with love, gratitude, and forgiveness	You'll feel better able to express love unconditionally and feel more compassion for all beings	Bija mantra: YAM Suggested asana: Supported fish
Solar plexus (*manipura* in Sanskrit)	Your relationship with yourself and is associated with self-esteem, willpower, and determination	You'll feel more confident, worthy of respect, and capable	Bija mantra: RAM Suggested asana: Lying spinal twist
Sacral (*svadhisthana* in Sanskrit)	Your relationships and emotions and is associated with sexuality and creativity	You'll feel more comfortable with your sexuality, more inspired, and more deeply connected to others	Bija mantra: VAM Suggested asana: Any dragon asana
Root (*muladhara* in Sanskrit)	Your ties to your culture and the physical world and is associated with safety, self-preservation, and survival	You'll feel more grounded, abundant, and secure	Bija mantra: LAM Suggested asanas: Deer or Squat

What are meridians?

In Chinese medicine, energy called *Qi* (pronounced "chee") flows through you in pathways called meridians. Keeping the meridians healthy and clear may increase longevity and support the proper function of your organs.

How meridians work

Meridians can be described as channels or pathways that control the flow of energy to and from various points in your body. They're not vessels in the physiological sense; they're more akin to energy paths that when clear might promote the efficient flow of energy through your body.

Liver	Gall bladder	Kidney	Bladder	Spleen	Stomach
Associated with: blood flow, tendon and ligament flexibility, and menstrual cycles	**Associated with:** bile and energy for movement and action	**Associated with:** sexual energy and the production of bone marrow	**Associated with:** the removal of liquid waste from the body	**Associated with:** digestion and the flow of nutrients in the body	**Associated with:** digestion and the mental state
When unbalanced: believed to cause stomach pain, back pain, stiffness in the joints, anger, and irritability	**When unbalanced:** believed to cause headaches, eye disorders, insomnia, timidity, and indecisiveness	**When unbalanced:** believed to cause urinary disorders, reproduction issues, back pain, fear, and insecurity	**When unbalanced:** believed to cause back pain, urinary disorders, vision problems, and indecisiveness	**When unbalanced:** believed to cause digestion issues, stomach problems, fatigue, brain fog, and excessive worry	**When unbalanced:** believed to cause digestion issues, stomach pain, excessive worry, and anxiety
Asana to help return you to balance: Straddle	**Asana to help return you to balance:** Banana	**Asana to help return you to balance:** Butterfly	**Asana to help return you to balance:** Caterpillar	**Asana to help return you to balance:** Saddle	**Asana to help return you to balance:** Twisted dragon

The 12 meridians and their asanas

It's believed that stress, difficulty processing emotions, and improper diet can block the meridians and immobilize the *Qi* flow in your body, causing physical problems or disease. The principles of this philosophy suggest that yin yoga might be ideal for helping to open up these blocked meridians, allowing *Qi* to flow more freely throughout your body, and bringing you more internal and external strength.

Practising the asanas in this book on a regular basis could help stimulate the meridians and allow your *Qi* to flow freely, nourishing your organs and replenishing your energy levels. By improving the health of your connective tissues and calming your mind and emotions through practice, you can allow *Qi* to flow more openly through your meridians. Whenever you feel out of balance, practising yin yoga might unblock your meridians.

Heart	Small intestine	Lung	Large intestine	Pericardium	Triple burner
Associated with: distributing blood to organs and governing emotions	**Associated with:** the separation of nutrients to be absorbed and eliminated	**Associated with:** the regulation of breath and the intake of energy	**Associated with:** the elimination of waste and the reabsorption of water	**Associated with:** the removal of excess energy and the protection of the heart	**Associated with:** the regulation of metabolism
When unbalanced: believed to cause chest pain, heart palpitations, sleep problems, anxiety, and depression	**When unbalanced:** believed to cause digestion issues, poor circulation, lower abdomen pain, and poor mental clarity	**When unbalanced:** believed to cause respiratory problems, throat and nose issues, sadness, and grief	**When unbalanced:** believed to cause constipation, sore throat, abdominal pain, worry, and difficulty letting go	**When unbalanced:** believed to cause heart problems, negative sexual feelings, and difficulty expressing emotions	**When unbalanced:** believed to cause appetite dysfunction, ear and throat problems, and emotional instability
Asana to help return you to balance: Sphinx	**Asana to help return you to balance:** Bowtie	**Asana to help return you to balance:** Melting heart	**Asana to help return you to balance:** Lying chest opener	**Asana to help return you to balance:** Wrist extensor stretch	**Asana to help return you to balance:** Eagle arms

Breathing techniques

Pranayama – the Sanskrit word for breathing exercises and controls – can help you balance your energy levels, facilitate a meditative state, and support your body during your yin yoga practice. Practising *pranayama* will help you slow down and deepen your breathing.

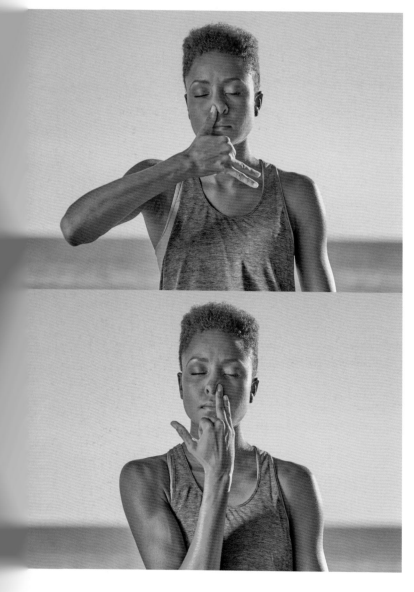

Alternate nostril breath

Perform the Alternate nostril breath – called *nadi shodan* in Sanskrit – before practising an asana, rather than during an asana. It can balance your energy levels and calm you down when you're overactive and stressed. You can even use this technique when not practising yin yoga.

1 Sit in a cross-legged position, with your hands resting on your thighs.

2 Lift your right hand up and bend your index and middle fingers towards your palm, bringing your right thumb to your right nostril and pressing to seal it shut.

3 Deeply inhale through your left nostril for a count of 4, 5, or 6.

4 Seal off your left nostril with your right ring finger and release your right nostril.

5 Exhale through your right nostril for the same count of 4, 5, or 6.

6 Deeply inhale through your right nostril for a count of 4, 5, or 6.

7 Seal off your right nostril with your right thumb and release your left nostril.

8 Exhale through your left nostril for the same count of 4, 5, or 6 to complete one round. Repeat these steps for 5 to 10 more rounds.

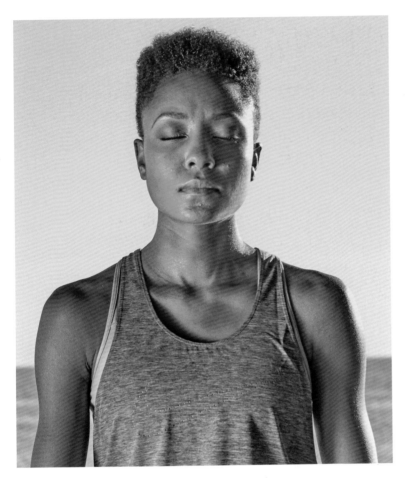

Ocean breath

The Ocean breath – called *ujjayi* in Sanskrit – is a breathing exercise you can do while performing yin yoga asanas. As you practise this technique, imagine you're trying to steam up a mirror with your breath, while keeping your mouth closed, breathing only through your nostrils. You should create a slight constriction at the back of your throat, which produces a soft sound similar to that of the ocean.

1 With a slight throat constriction, inhale through your nose for a count of 4, 5, or 6.

2 Pause at the top of the inhale for a count of 1.

3 With a slight throat constriction, exhale through your nose for a count of 4, 5, or 6.

4 Pause at the end of the exhale for a count of 1 to complete one round. Repeat these steps for 5 to 10 rounds.

Humming bee breath

Performing Humming bee breath – called *bhramari* in Sanskrit – is best done before practising an asana. This simple breathing exercise can help calm your nerves and quieten a busy mind.

1 Sit in a cross-legged position, with your hands resting on your thighs.

2 Press your index fingers to the cartilage between your cheek and ear to block outside noise, keeping your elbows lifted.

3 Inhale a deep breath through your nose.

4 Exhale through your nose while making a long "mmmmm" sound aloud – like a bee buzzing – to complete one round. Repeat these steps for 3 to 5 rounds.

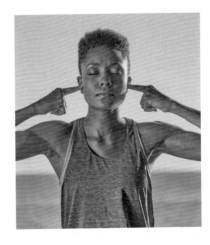

What do you need?

Props are essential components of a yin yoga practice and allow you to perform yin asanas more safely and effectively. The most commonly used yin yoga props discussed here are featured throughout this book.

Blocks

Blocks are used to fill the gaps between your body and the ground and to provide support for your body during more challenging postures.

What to buy: Blocks come in wood, cork, foam, and bamboo, giving you several different options for comfort and budget. It's best to have two blocks on hand for your yin yoga practice. You can also use large – but firm – cushions or pillows.

Bolsters

Bolsters are large yoga cushions that are useful for providing support during more difficult positions. Bolsters provide you with a more stable surface that you can lie back on or use to prop yourself up comfortably, which will help you hold postures for extended periods of time.

What to buy: Choose a large rectangular or cylindrical bolster that's roughly the length of your spine. You can also use a dense sofa cushion or pillow.

Yoga blankets

Yoga blankets provide extra padding for your hands and knees, especially if you have a thinner mat. They also can be used to provide comfort and support to your legs when you're sitting cross-legged and need to elevate your hips.

What to buy: Cotton is your best bet, but you can use any thick blankets you already own.

Straps

Straps help you extend your reach if you have limited flexibility. They'll also help you gain stability and perform reclining asanas more efficiently.

What to buy: Most yoga straps are between 1.75 to 3 metres (6 to 10ft) long. Choose one that feels comfortable between your hands. You can also use a belt or a length of soft rope.

Mats

A yoga mat is used to provide comfort and keep your body off the surface below you. It will also help you to maintain balance.

What to buy: Consider thickness when buying a yoga mat. Standard mats are usually 3mm (⅛in) thick, but if you have sensitive joints, a mat that's 6mm (¼in) thick will provide additional support. If you haven't got a mat, use a blanket.

How do you practise?

Reaping the full benefits of yin yoga requires you to hold postures for extended periods of time. This section will help ensure that your body and mind are prepared for a complete yin experience.

How and when to practise

Make the most of your yin yoga practice by creating an environment in which you have the physical space and the time for an effective and consistent yin yoga experience.

Find a quiet, peaceful space
Choose a space that's free of distractions. Maintaining a home yoga practice means making the time you spend on your mat feel like a retreat from the stresses of everyday life. Your peaceful space doesn't have to be luxurious nor does it need to be indoors, but you should feel safe and protected from distractions – electronic or otherwise.

Set the mood You can set the mood for a more meditative atmosphere by playing soft ambient music in the background, lighting a few candles, or using essential oils.

Lay out your props To prevent the need to pause after you've started, have all the props that you will need for that day's asanas laid out around you before you begin.

Practise with cold muscles
Practising when your muscles are cold helps to emphasize the strengthening and lengthening of the connective tissues,

as opposed to the muscles. This means you don't need to perform any warm-ups.

Refrain from eating Avoid eating a meal right before practice. Give your body a few hours to digest food beforehand, so you'll feel comfortable in the postures.

Start your experience slowly
If you're new to yin yoga, start by practising once or twice a week and increase this if your body allows it, ensuring you take at least one full day's rest every week. And make sure you start each practice with the seated meditation (see page 24).

Using this book

This book is made up of asanas and sequences. Asanas are individual postures, and sequences are a series of asanas targeting a specific goal.

The asanas Each asana includes step-by-step instructions for effectively performing the posture. Read through every step before attempting a posture, including any modifications. Listen to your body and change the hold times depending on how you feel. Be sure to take note of any physical concerns or limitations included with each asana, so you can perform each one safely.

The asana's effects   Step-by-step instructions

Points to be aware of   Modifications

Practice early or late An early morning session can awaken your body and mind for the day ahead. It can also help loosen up joints that are stiff from a night of sleep. A session just before bedtime can place your mind and body in a restful state and prepare you for a better night's sleep. Practise yin yoga when it feels right for you.

Plan ahead Set time aside for your practice – whether every day or every other day. Remember that you'll be holding postures for long periods of time, so you won't be doing too many asanas during a 30-minute session. Also remember to include time for any breathing exercises you might want to do.

End every session in Corpse pose Resting in the Corpse pose for a few minutes at the end of your practice will give your mind and body an opportunity to fully integrate the work you've done during the practice.

Total time for the sequence

Which asanas to practise

Required props

Suggested hold time

The sequences In addition to individual asanas, there are 20 sequences – which group specific asanas together – with total hold times ranging from 30 to 90 minutes. Before starting a selected sequence, read through all the asanas and ensure you have all necesssary props nearby. You can modify sequences to suit your needs by changing the hold times of the asanas, adding or removing meditations or breathing techniques, or performing the "Make it easier" or "Make it harder" options for an asana.

Seated meditation

Begin your yin yoga practice with the seated meditation, which will help ease you into a meditative state before practising the postures in this book. Finding a restful, meditative state is as easy as following a few steps – with the goal being to gradually lengthen the spaces between thoughts.

How to meditate

Meditation is a simple process, but the benefits are immeasurable. Before you begin, try to find a peaceful, quiet location that's free of any distractions.

1 Sit in a comfortable seated position. Place your hands on your thighs or knees, straighten your back, and extend the crown of your head upwards.

2 Close your eyes and visualize yourself in a peaceful place. Focus on the sensations you might feel – such as a light breeze on your face or the sound of running water – as if you were there.

3 Imagine your body being surrounded by a warm, radiant white light.

4 Inhale slow, steady breaths through your nose and imagine yourself breathing in the light.

5 Allow your body and mind to relax as you exhale slowly through your nose. Remain in this position for as long as desired.

Helpful hints

- If you notice discomfort in your hips or lower back, sit on a block or a folded blanket for support.

- If you feel your muscles tightening up, bring your awareness back to your breathing and focus on relaxing your muscles with every exhale.

- If you're struggling with a recurring negative thought or emotion, imagine inhaling a calm feeling and expelling the negative thought or emotion with each exhale.

- If you want to achieve an even deeper level of relaxation, internally repeat a *bija* (mantra) as you inhale deeply through your nose and again for the duration of your exhale.

Extend the crown
of your head upwards

Close your eyes and soften
the muscles around your
eyes and mouth

Drop your shoulders away from
your ears, continuing to keep your
back straight, and allow gravity to
pull your tailbone into the ground

Sit on the ground in a comfortable
position, crossing your legs and
keeping your tailbone on the ground

Place your hands
on your knees

Yin asanas

Within this chapter you'll discover more than 50 yoga postures – each designed to be held for an extended period. These asanas were created with one goal: to offer a life-changing impact on your body *and* your mind.

Square

This asana stretches your lower back, helps reinforce outer hip rotation (which can help alleviate knee strain), and could help promote healthy digestion by compressing your stomach.

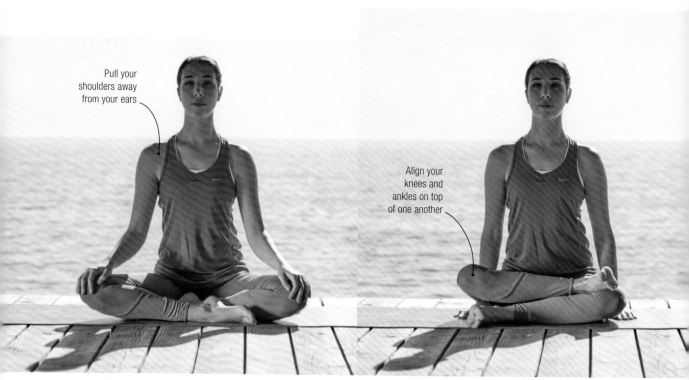

Pull your shoulders away from your ears

Align your knees and ankles on top of one another

1 Sit on the ground in a comfortable position, crossing your legs and keeping your tailbone on the ground. Put your hands on your knees and extend the crown of your head upwards.

2 Place your right foot on your left knee and tuck your left foot under your right knee. Flex your feet so your toes point towards your knees.

BE AWARE If you have sciatica or knee pain, or have ever suffered lower back or knee injuries, you should avoid this posture, since it might aggravate these conditions.

*Allow any distractions
to drift into the background –
stay present*

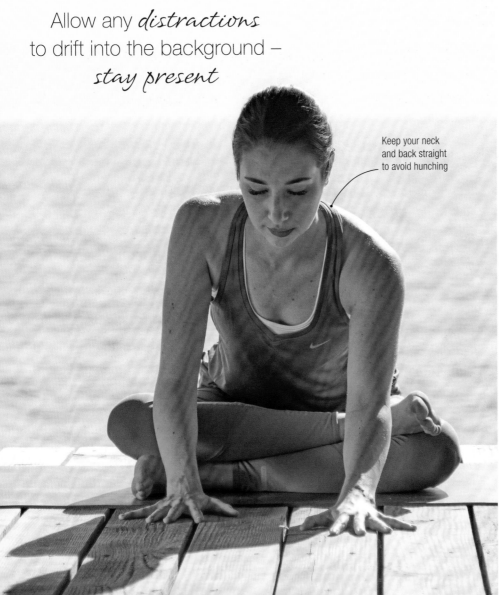

Keep your neck
and back straight
to avoid hunching

MAKE IT EASIER
In step 2, place
blocks under
your knees and
put your hands
behind you.

MAKE IT HARDER
In step 3, place
your hands further
away from your
body and rest
your forehead
and forearms
on the ground.

3 Lean forwards from your hips and slide your hands forwards
until you find your edge, but don't go all the way to the ground.
Hold. Inhale and exhale slow, steady breaths through your nose.
Slowly reverse out of the posture.

Reclining leg stretch 1

This asana opens up your entire leg – from hamstring to ankle – providing a full lower body stretch without putting excess stress on your lower back. You'll need a strap for this posture.

Keep your shoulder blades flat on the ground

1 Lie on your back and bend your knees, keeping your feet flat on the ground. Relax your arms at your sides and hold the strap in your right hand.

2 Transfer one end of the strap to your left hand and bring your right knee towards your chest. Slip the strap around the ball of your right foot.

BE AWARE If you've ever suffered hamstring injuries or tears, you should avoid this posture, or use caution by keeping your extended leg slightly bent at the knee.

Extend the toes of your left foot towards your left knee

3 Extend your right leg upwards while extending your left leg until it's flat on the ground. Pull your shoulders towards the ground and lightly pull on the strap to bring your right foot closer to your head, without bending your knee. **Hold.** Inhale and exhale slow, steady breaths through your nose. Slowly reverse out of the posture as you return to your starting position, then repeat with the opposite leg.

MAKE IT EASIER
In step 3, keep both knees slightly bent.

Reclining leg stretch 2

This asana cultivates deep flexibility in your inner groin and hamstrings, while allowing the upper back to relax. It can also help restore energy to the body. You'll need a strap for this posture.

Keep your shoulder blades flat on the ground

1 Lie on your back and bend your knees, keeping your feet flat on the ground. Relax your arms at your sides and hold the strap in your right hand.

2 Transfer one end of the strap to your left hand and bring your right knee towards your chest. Slip the strap around the ball of your right foot.

BE AWARE If you feel pain in your neck or upper back, place a blanket or pillow under your head to help your neck and upper back remain comfortable.

Extend the toes of your left foot towards your left knee

Keep both hips square to the mat

3 Extend your right leg upwards while extending your left leg until it's flat on the ground. Pull your shoulders towards the ground and lightly pull the strap to bring your right leg closer to your head, without bending your knee.

4 Transfer both ends of the strap to your right hand and extend your left arm so that it's perpendicular to your body. Keep your left arm and your shoulder blades flat on the ground.

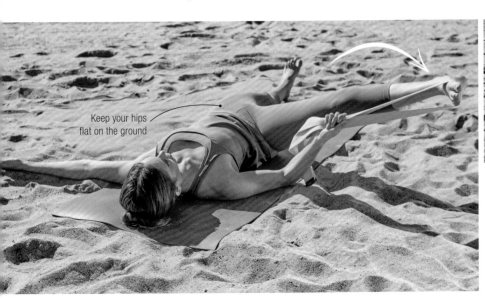

Keep your hips flat on the ground

MAKE IT EASIER
In step 5, bend your left knee, but keep your left foot flat on the ground. You can also place a bolster under your right thigh.

5 Keep your right leg fully extended as you lightly pull your right leg so that it's almost parallel to your left arm. **Hold.** Inhale and exhale slow, steady breaths through your nose. Slowly reverse out of the posture as you return to your starting position, then repeat with the opposite leg.

Reclining leg stretch 3

This twisting asana – which can stretch your chest and help relieve lower back pain – encourages healthy digestion and offers a deep leg stretch. You'll need a strap for this posture.

Keep your shoulder blades flat on the ground

1 Lie on your back and bend your knees, keeping your feet flat on the ground. Relax your arms at your sides and hold a strap in your right hand.

2 Transfer one end of the strap to your left hand and bring your left knee towards your chest. Slip the strap around the ball of your left foot.

BE AWARE If you've ever suffered slipped or herniated discs, you should avoid this posture, since it could aggravate these conditions.

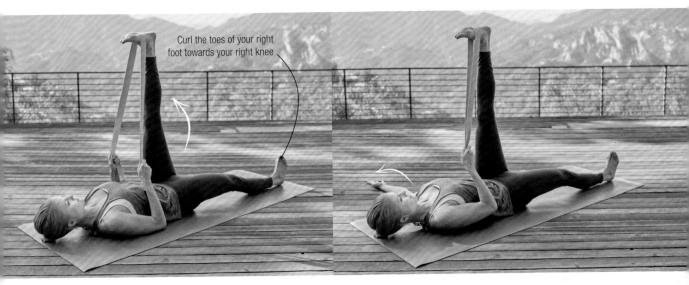

Curl the toes of your right foot towards your right knee

3 Extend your left leg upwards while extending your right leg until it's flat on the ground. Continue to keep your head, shoulder blades, and right heel flat on the ground.

4 Transfer both ends of the strap to your right hand. Extend your left arm until it's perpendicular to your body, keeping it flat on the ground, with your left palm facing up.

MAKE IT EASIER
In step 5, support your twisting leg with a block or a bolster.

5 Cross your left leg over your right leg, making your left leg parallel to your left arm. **Hold.** Inhale and exhale slow, steady breaths through your nose. Slowly reverse out of the posture as you return to your starting position, then repeat with the opposite leg.

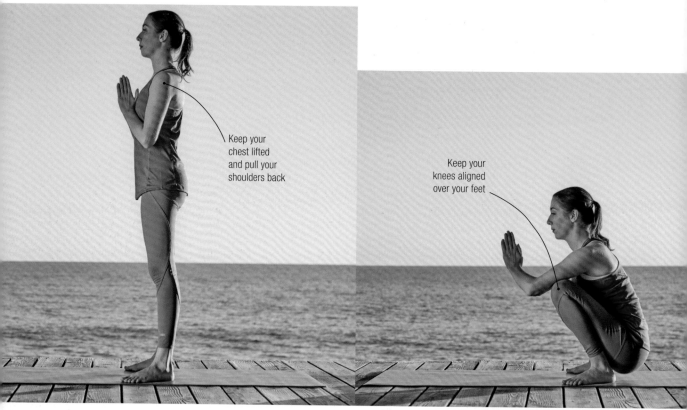

Keep your
chest lifted
and pull your
shoulders back

Keep your
knees aligned
over your feet

1 Stand with your feet hip-width apart.
Turn your feet out so that your toes point
towards the top corners of the mat and place
your hands in a praying position at your heart.

2 Bend your knees to lower your hips
towards the ground. Your hips should
hover off the ground and your feet should
remain flat on the ground.

Squat

This soothing and stabilizing asana helps with outer
hip rotation and opens up your lower back. Staying in a
low position can help you attain the grounded feelings –
physically and mentally – you need for balance in your life.

BE AWARE Although this asana can strengthen your ankles, if you've ever suffered any kind of
ankle injury, use caution with this posture, or perform the Reclined child's pose (page 120) instead.

Push your knees as wide open as possible

Tap into the *grounding nature* of this posture by feeling your energy take root in your *feet*

3 Rest your elbows on the inside of your thighs and use your arms to press your knees open. Extend the crown of your head upwards and lengthen your tailbone to elongate your spine. **Hold.** Inhale and exhale slow, steady breaths through your nose. Slowly reverse out of the posture.

MAKE IT EASIER
In step 2, place a block under your hips for elevation. You can also place a rolled-up blanket under your heels if they're lifting off the ground.

Toe squat

This asana targets your lower legs – an area often neglected by traditional exercise. Having flexible feet will help you maintain a strong foundation for balance and agility.

Spread your toes wide

1 Put your hands and knees flat on the ground, pointing your fingers forwards. Keep your spine and neck parallel to the ground and your eyes looking down.

2 Flex your feet and curl your toes towards your knees, keeping your toes flat on the ground. Shift your body back to centre your hips over your heels, continuing to align your neck and back.

BE AWARE While this asana stretches the toes and soles of your feet, if you've got weak knees or ankles, you might find this posture uncomfortable or difficult to hold.

Visualize a current of *energy* drawing up from your toes to the *crown of your head*

Keep your back and neck straight

3 Continue to shift your hips back to rest them on your heels. Place your palms on your thighs. **Hold.** Inhale and exhale slow, steady breaths through your nose. Slowly reverse out of the posture.

MAKE IT EASIER
In step 3, keep your hips slightly elevated and put your hands on the ground in front of you, using only your fingers for support.

IT band stretch

Runners will appreciate this hip-opening asana that targets the legs, from your hips to your knees. In this area are your iliotibial (IT) bands – the connective tissues that extend from your pelvic bone to your shinbone – which are difficult to target and thus easy to neglect.

Keep your head and shoulder blades flat on the ground

1 Lie on your back and bend your knees, relaxing your arms at your sides and keeping your feet and hands flat on the ground. Relax your neck and look straight up towards the sky.

2 Slowly raise your right foot over your left knee and rest your right ankle just above your left knee. Extend your right toes upwards to relieve tension on your right knee and gently push your right knee away from your body.

BE AWARE Although this posture can help with post-workout recovery, use caution if you have IT band syndrome, since overstretching the IT band can aggravate the problem.

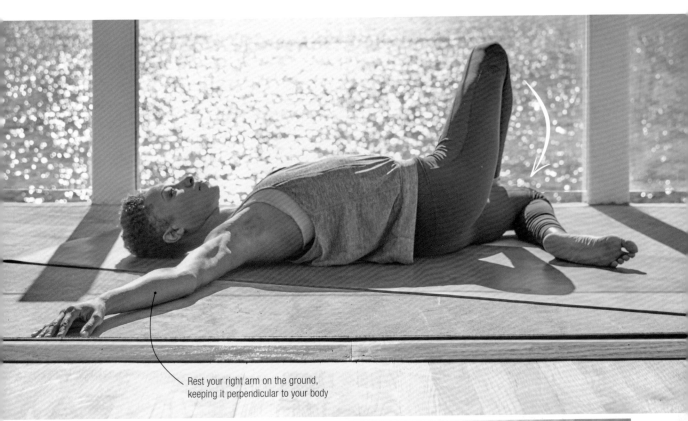

Rest your right arm on the ground, keeping it perpendicular to your body

3 Rotate your hips to lower your left thigh and right foot towards the ground on your left side, until your right foot makes contact with the ground. Grab your right ankle with your left hand. **Hold.** Inhale and exhale slow, steady breaths through your nose. Slowly reverse out of the posture as you return to your starting position, then repeat with the opposite leg.

MAKE IT EASIER
In step 3, place a block under the foot of the crossing leg.

Neck release

Neck tension is one of the most common complaints people have. Taking a few minutes to stretch this area can help you release stress and improve your posture.

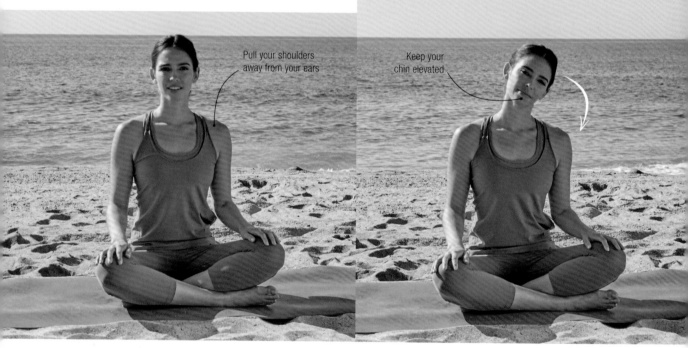

Pull your shoulders
away from your ears

Keep your
chin elevated

1 Sit on the ground in a comfortable position, crossing your legs and keeping your tailbone on the ground. Put your hands on your knees and extend the crown of your head upwards.

2 Drop your left ear towards your left shoulder without letting your chin drop to your chest. Keep your shoulders level and aligned over your hips and let your head become heavy so your neck can relax.

BE AWARE If you've ever suffered a cervical spine injury, you can tilt your head in a different direction or just avoid this posture entirely.

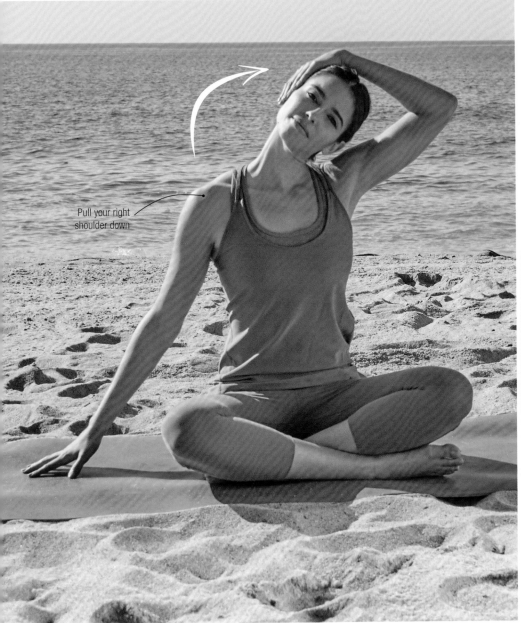

Pull your right
shoulder down

MAKE IT EASIER
In step 3, put your
hand behind your
right ear and let
your chin tilt down
towards your
left shoulder.

3 Reach your right arm out to your right side, putting your fingertips
on the ground, and curl your left hand over your head to place
it over your right ear. Pull your head further away from your right
shoulder. **Hold.** Inhale and exhale slow, steady breaths through your
nose. Slowly reverse out of the posture as you return to your starting
position, then repeat on the opposite side.

Point your
toes away
from you

Keep
your spine
straight

1 Sit in a kneeling position, allowing your hips
to sit on your heels. Rest your palms on
your thighs and extend the crown of your
head upwards.

2 Reach your arms behind you, putting
your fingers on the ground for support,
and pointing them away from you as you
shift your weight back onto your feet.

Ankle stretch

If you have problems kneeling or squatting, this asana can help
improve flexibility in your ankles, allowing you to perform these
types of movements more easily.

BE AWARE This is a simple but intense stretch, so if you find this posture uncomfortable
or difficult to hold, or if you have inflexible ankles, use a blanket for balance support.

Focus on your *breathing* rather than continually trying to *maintain* your balance

Lift your chest and use your arms for extra balance support

3 Lift your knees and shins off the ground, continuing to use your fingers for support. **Hold.** Inhale and exhale slow, steady breaths through your nose. Slowly reverse out of the posture.

MAKE IT EASIER
In step 3, place a block under your hips and a folded blanket under your knees.

MAKE IT HARDER
In step 3, go deeper into the posture by putting your palms on your knees while still lifting your shins off the ground. Use your core strength to help you stay balanced.

"Yoga is the practice of *quieting the mind*"

Patanjali

Caterpillar

This asana provides a full-body stretch – ideal for relaxation and eliminating stress. It might also help with digestion, because the forward fold compresses your stomach.

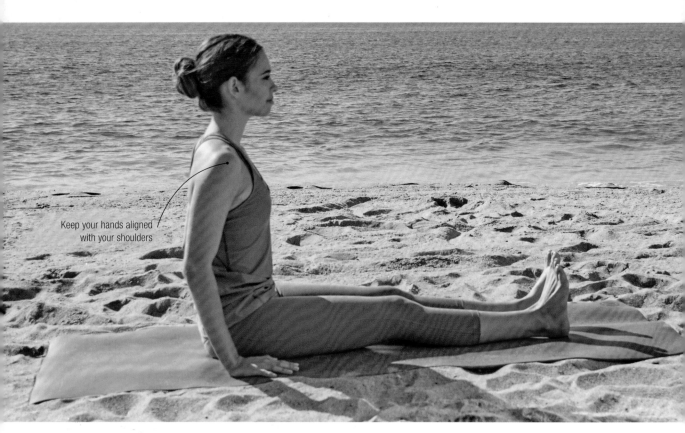

Keep your hands aligned with your shoulders

1 Sit up tall, stretching your legs out in front of you and placing your hands on the ground at your sides. Keep your tailbone on the ground and extend the crown of your head upwards.

BE AWARE This asana can stretch the muscles around your spine. If you have sciatica, performing this posture could aggravate the condition.

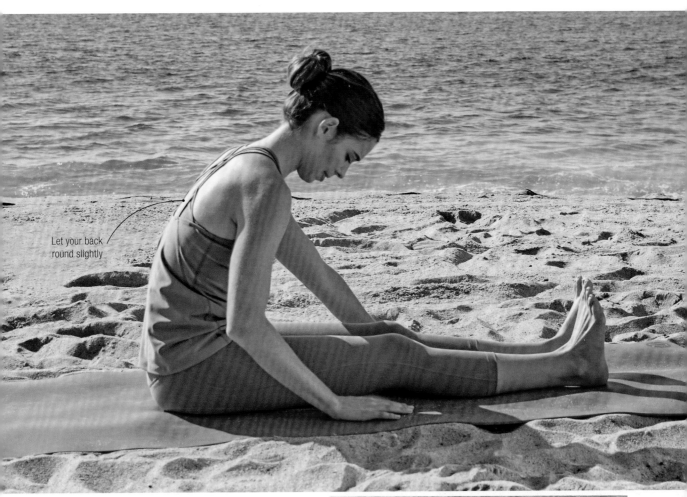

Let your back
round slightly

2 Walk your hands towards your knees and tilt your pelvis forwards until you find your edge. Relax your head, neck, and arms, letting gravity do the work. Slightly bend your knees to prevent them locking up. **Hold.** Inhale and exhale slow, steady breaths through your nose. Slowly reverse out of the posture.

MAKE IT EASIER
In step 1, sit on a block to help your pelvis tilt forwards. You can also place a bolster between your chest and legs for more support, or add a smaller bolster under your knees to keep them bent.

Butterfly

This seated asana provides one of the best stretches for your inner groin, while also improving hip flexibility and stretching your lower back. It is also thought to help improve kidney and prostate functions.

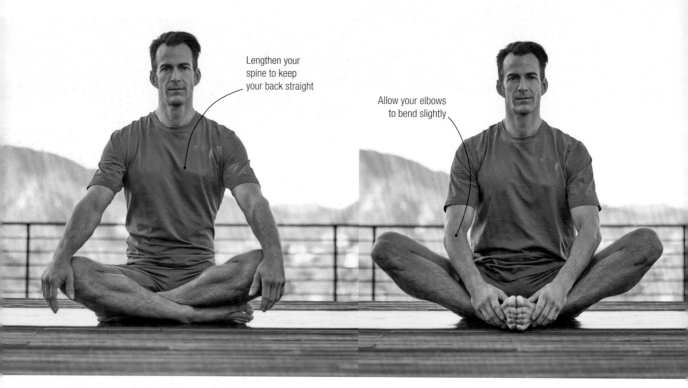

Lengthen your spine to keep your back straight

Allow your elbows to bend slightly

1 Sit on the ground in a comfortable position, crossing your legs and keeping your tailbone on the ground. Put your hands on your knees and extend the crown of your head upwards.

2 Bring the soles of your feet together and use your hands to pull your heels closer to your groin.

BE AWARE If you have sciatica, use caution when performing this posture, since it can aggravate the condition.

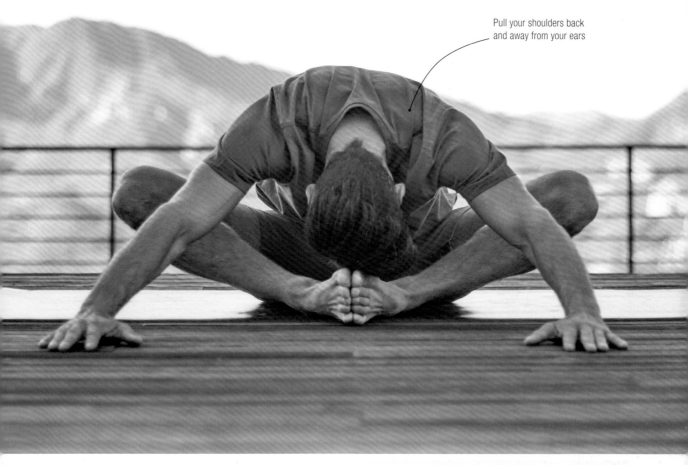

Pull your shoulders back and away from your ears

3 Fold forwards from your hips, letting gravity take over until you find your edge. Place your hands out wide in front of you, keeping your palms flat on the ground. Relax your neck and slightly round your spine. **Hold.** Inhale and exhale slow, steady breaths through your nose. Slowly reverse out of the posture.

MAKE IT EASIER
In step 3, elevate your hips by sitting on a folded blanket or a bolster.

Half butterfly

This asana opens your hips through outer hip rotation and stretches deeply into your hamstrings. The forward fold lightly compresses your internal organs, promoting healthy digestion.

Lengthen your spine to keep your back straight

Keep your toes pointing upwards

1 Sit on the ground in a comfortable position, crossing your legs and keeping your tailbone on the ground. Put your hands on your knees and extend the crown of your head upwards.

2 Extend your right leg out to the side and bend your left knee to place the sole of your left foot on the inside of your right thigh.

BE AWARE If you have limited hamstring flexibility or have ever suffered a hamstring injury, this posture could cause significant discomfort, so keep a gentle bend in your knees.

Keep your back straight and your spine aligned

3 Turn your upper body towards your right leg, put your hands on the ground to either side of your right leg, and slowly walk your hands forwards, pressing your left thigh down to keep your tailbone on the ground.

4 Let your upper body relax and your back round as you fold your stomach towards your right thigh until you find your edge. **Hold.** Inhale and exhale slow, steady breaths through your nose. Slowly reverse out of the posture as you return to your starting position, then repeat with the opposite leg.

MAKE IT EASIER
In step 4, walk your hands out in front of your hips – rather than turning to the side – and place a block or a bolster under your forehead for support.

Reclined butterfly

This asana is a restorative way to open up your hips and stretch your inner groin, as well as improving hip flexibility. Although this posture is mostly passive, it's also intense, so ensure you're in a comfortable position throughout.

1 Lie on your back, keeping your legs and shoulder blades flat on the ground and relaxing your arms at your sides, with your palms facing up.

BE AWARE This posture requires little effort, but it can put a strain on weakened or injured knees, so place blankets or blocks under your knees to help relieve any discomfort.

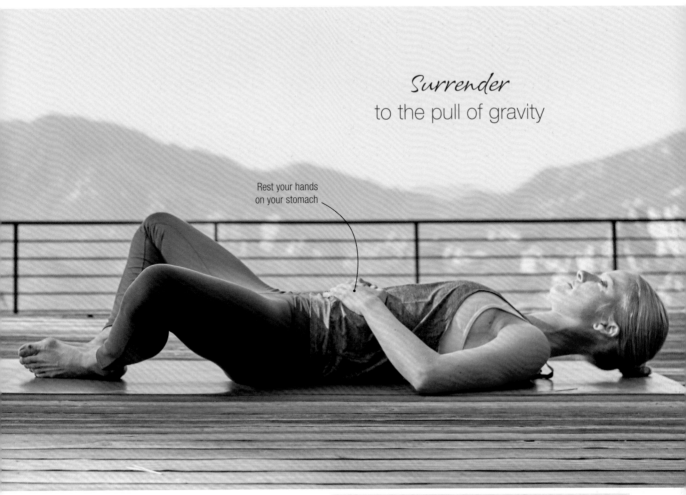

Surrender
to the pull of gravity

Rest your hands
on your stomach

2 Bend your knees so the soles of your feet
touch. Bring your heels closer to your groin,
and relax your legs to let gravity pull them
towards the ground. **Hold.** Inhale and exhale
slow, steady breaths through your nose.
Slowly reverse out of the posture.

MAKE IT EASIER
In step 2, place a block under each thigh.

Align your elbow
with your shoulder

1 Lie on your stomach, stack your palms under your forehead, and fully extend your legs behind you.

2 Reach your left arm out to the side, bending your elbow at a 90-degree angle and keeping your left palm flat on the ground.

Lying chest opener

This energizing asana helps counteract the excessive shoulder hunching you do while driving or sitting at a desk. It also improves overall posture and shoulder flexibility while requiring minimal effort.

BE AWARE If you feel a tingling sensation down either arm while performing this asana, carefully reverse your movements to slowly back out of the posture.

3 Reach your right arm out to your side, bend your right elbow, and place your right hand flat on the ground next to your ribcage.

Internally say "I surrender" on your *inhale* and "I let go" on your *exhale*

Pull your shoulders away from your ears

4 Slowly push your right hand into the ground to lift your right side up, and roll onto your left ear, shoulder, and hip. Bend your knees slightly and allow your legs to relax, keeping them stacked. **Hold.** Inhale and exhale slow, steady breaths through your nose. Slowly reverse out of the posture as you return to your starting position, then repeat on the opposite side.

MAKE IT EASIER
In step 4, place a block under your head.

MAKE IT HARDER
In step 4, place the back of the hand of your top arm on your lower back and extend your top leg behind you.

Lying quad stretch

This simple asana opens up your upper legs and can help you prepare for doing backbends. If you're a runner, you'll find this posture beneficial for relieving muscular aches and pains in your thighs. It can also reduce post-workout leg stiffness.

Place your legs hip-width apart

Keep your chest flat on the ground

1 Lie on your stomach, stack your hands under your forehead, and fully extend your legs behind you, keeping your toes flat on the ground and your neck and back straight.

2 Bend your right knee to bring your right leg towards your head, and reach your right hand behind you to grab the outer side of your right foot.

BE AWARE If you've ever suffered any lower back injury, use a strap to help make this posture more comfortable.

3 Gently pull your right foot towards your glutes and extend your tailbone towards your feet to lengthen the lower back. **Hold.** Inhale and exhale slow, steady breaths through your nose. Slowly reverse out of the posture as you return to your starting position, then repeat with the opposite leg.

MAKE IT EASIER
In step 3, use a strap around the top of the foot of the bent leg.

1 Lie on your back and bend your knees, keeping your feet flat on the ground. Place your arms at your sides to create 90-degree angles, with your palms facing up.

2 Press your feet down into the ground and slide your hips a few inches to your right. Continue keeping your head and shoulder blades flat on the ground.

Lying spinal twist

Supine twists offer a gentle compression of the stomach, which may help improve digestion. This particular twist can also stretch your lower back, helping with mobility.

BE AWARE Although twists might soothe back pain, you should avoid them if you've suffered any kind of spinal injury.

Keep your shoulder
blades and head
on the ground

3 Anchoring your right shoulder blade to the ground, let both legs drop down to your left until your left leg is flat on the ground. **Hold.** Inhale and exhale slow, steady breaths through your nose. Slowly reverse out of the posture as you return to your starting position, then repeat on the opposite side.

MAKE IT EASIER
In step 3, place a block under your knees.

MAKE IT HARDER
In step 3, cross your top thigh over your bottom thigh – but don't alter the position of your shoulders.

Saddle

This asana opens up the front of your thighs and stretches your ankle and knee joints through inner hip rotation. It will also stretch your quadriceps, hip flexors, and shoulders for a full-body experience.

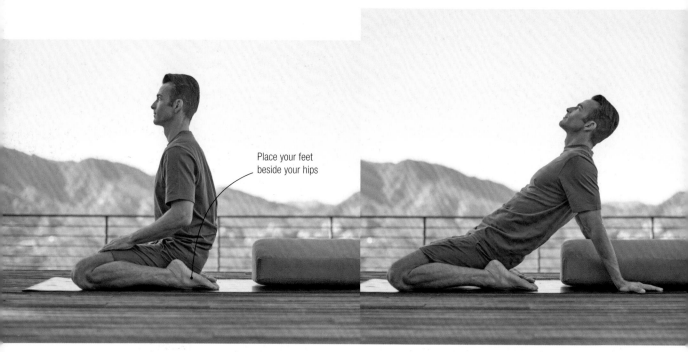

Place your feet beside your hips

1 Place a bolster behind you. Sit in a kneeling position, placing your legs outside your hips, and keep your tailbone on the ground. Keep the tops of your feet flat on the ground and point your toes straight back. Lengthen your spine and rest your palms on your thighs.

2 Extend your arms behind you and walk your hands towards the bolster. Extend your tailbone towards your heels to lengthen your lower back and keep your legs flat on the ground. Keep your back and neck straight as you begin to lower yourself onto the bolster behind you.

BE AWARE If you feel pain in your knees and ankles, or have suffered any knee or ankle injuries, use a blanket or a bolster for support.

Visualize a *radiating* white light
at the centre of your *heart*

Keep your
knees touching
the ground

3 Lower all the way down to the bolster (or go all the way to the ground) and extend your arms over your head to stretch your chest and shoulders. **Hold.** Inhale and exhale slow, steady breaths through your nose. Slowly reverse out of the posture.

MAKE IT EASIER
In step 3, put a blanket and a block behind your thighs and on top of the backs of your calves to keep your hips elevated. Walk your hands behind you and hold yourself up.

Archer arms

This asana encourages deep breathing by opening up your chest and improving flexibility in your shoulders. You'll also feel your upper arms and upper back stretch and strengthen.

Lengthen your spine to keep your back straight

1 Sit on the ground in a comfortable position, crossing your legs and keeping your tailbone on the ground. Put your hands on your knees and extend the crown of your head upwards.

2 Reach your right arm over your right shoulder, bend your right elbow, and place your fingers below your neck, between your shoulders.

BE AWARE If you've suffered any kind of shoulder injury, this posture might aggravate it. You might find that using a strap helps alleviate some discomfort.

Feel your ribcage *expand* from front to back and side to side as you *breathe in and out* through your nose

Pull your elbows away from one another to keep your chest open

MAKE IT EASIER
In step 3, hold a strap in both hands.

3 Reach your left arm behind your back, bend your left elbow, and reach your left hand up to your right hand to interlace your fingers. **Hold.** Inhale and exhale slow, steady breaths through your nose. Slowly reverse out of the posture as you return to your starting position, then switch arm positions and repeat.

"*Conscious breathing* is my anchor"

Thich Nhat Hanh

Keep your shoulder blades
flat on the ground

1 Lie on your back and extend your legs straight
out in front of you, with your feet hip-width apart.

Knee to chest

This hip-opening asana gently stretches your lower back and
compresses your stomach to encourage healthy digestion. You
can practise this posture as a morning warm-up or before bed.

BE AWARE If you've ever suffered any kind of spinal or knee injury,
use caution when performing this asana.

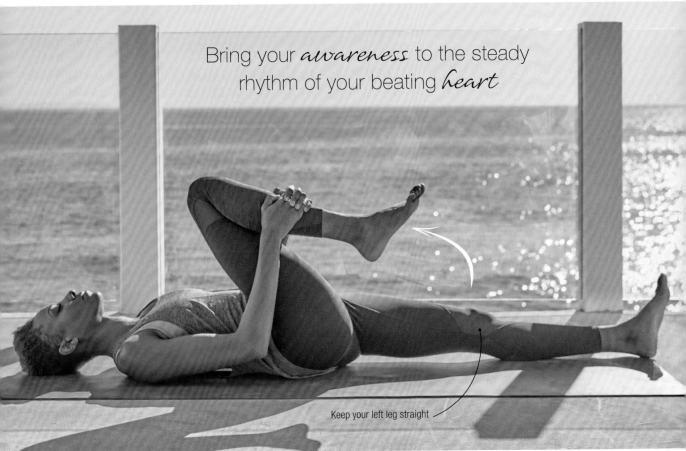

Bring your *awareness* to the steady
rhythm of your beating *heart*

Keep your left leg straight

2 Wrap your hands around your right shin
and pull your right knee into your chest.
Press down through your left heel to keep
your left leg extended, and soften your
shoulders, keeping them in contact with
the ground. **Hold.** Inhale and exhale slow,
steady breaths through your nose. Slowly
reverse out of the posture as you return
to your starting position, then repeat with
the opposite leg.

MAKE IT EASIER
In step 2, bend your left knee and keep your left
foot flat on the ground as you pull your right knee
towards your stomach.

Keep your elbows straight

1 Put your hands and knees on the ground, with your hands flat and your fingers pointing forwards. Keep your spine and neck parallel to the ground and your eyes looking down.

2 Rotate your right hand clockwise, so that your fingertips point towards your right knee. Spread your fingers wide to keep your weight evenly distributed through your hands.

Wrist flexor stretch

This simple stretch will free up your wrists and forearms and soothe aching joints, especially if you suffer from carpal tunnel syndrome.

BE AWARE If you've ever suffered any kind of wrist injury, you might want to avoid this stretch. Go slowly – and stop if you experience any pain.

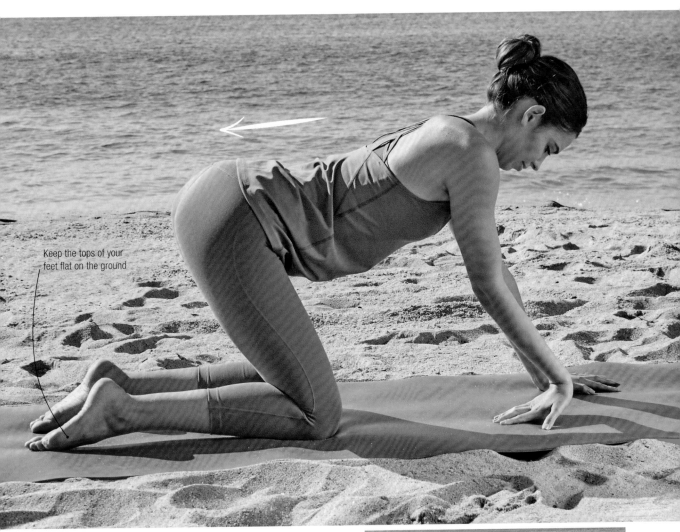

Keep the tops of your feet flat on the ground

3 Slowly shift your weight back towards your heels and lift your right palm off the ground, keeping your fingertips and your left hand flat on the ground. **Hold.** Inhale and exhale slow, steady breaths through your nose. Slowly reverse out of the posture as you return to your starting position, then repeat with the opposite hand.

MAKE IT EASIER
In step 2, rotate your fingers towards the outer edge of the mat.

Wrist extensor stretch

This asana will help improve your wrist mobility and deeply stretch your forearms. It is especially beneficial if you suffer from tennis elbow.

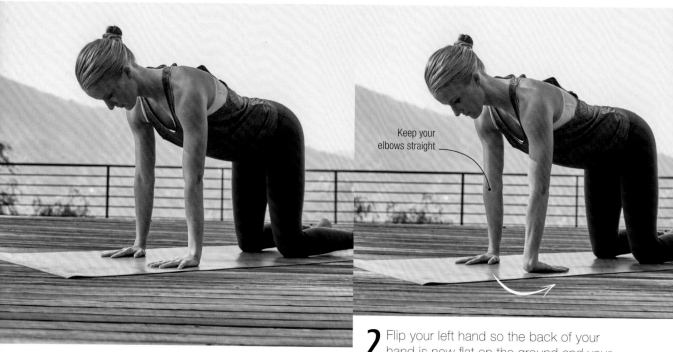

Keep your elbows straight

1 Put your hands and knees on the ground, with your hands flat and your fingers pointing forwards. Keep your spine and neck parallel to the ground and your eyes looking down.

2 Flip your left hand so the back of your hand is now flat on the ground and your fingertips point towards your left knee. Spread your fingers wide and keep your weight evenly distributed through your hands.

BE AWARE If you've ever suffered any kind of wrist injury, you might want to avoid this stretch. Go slowly – and stop if you experience any pain.

Lengthen your spine
to keep your back straight

Allow your thumb
to lift naturally

3 Slowly shift your weight back towards your heels
and lift the back of your left hand off the ground,
while keeping your knuckles and your right hand
flat on the ground. **Hold.** Inhale and exhale slow,
steady breaths through your nose. Slowly reverse
out of the posture as you return to your starting
position, then repeat with the opposite hand.

MAKE IT EASIER
In step 2, rotate your fingers towards the
centre of the mat after flipping your hand.

Sphinx

This heart-opening asana will help you learn to breathe deeply into your chest and upper back, while providing a backbend that can help reduce lower back pain and improve spine flexibility.

Relax your neck

1 Lie on your stomach, bending your elbows at 90-degree angles and stacking your hands in front of your head. Keep your hands and forearms flat on the ground. Rest your forehead on the ground and extend your legs fully behind you.

BE AWARE If you've ever suffered any kind of back injury, use caution when doing backbends. Go slowly – and stop if you experience any pain.

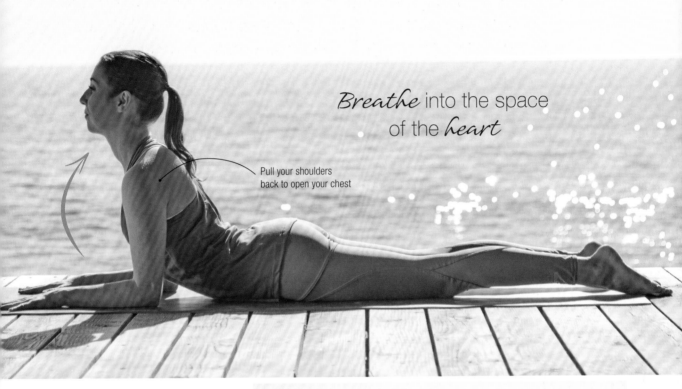

Breathe into the space of the *heart*

Pull your shoulders back to open your chest

2 Press your forearms into the ground and slide your hands back to lift up your head and chest. Align your elbows with your shoulders and spread your fingers wide. Extend your tailbone towards your heels and pull your chest forwards, relaxing your upper body as much as possible. **Hold.** Inhale and exhale slow, steady breaths through your nose. Slowly reverse out of the posture.

MAKE IT EASIER
In step 2, slide your arms further forwards.

1 Lie on your stomach, bending your elbows and keeping your hands and forearms flat on the ground in front of you. Press your forearms into the ground to lift your chest and head, and fully extend your legs behind you.

Seal

This asana is similar to the Sphinx, but it provides a much deeper backbend and could also help improve digestion. This is a great posture to do if you spend long hours sitting in a chair, because it reinforces the natural curve of your lower back.

BE AWARE If you experience pain in your lower back or sacrum while performing this posture, perform the Sphinx (page 74) instead.

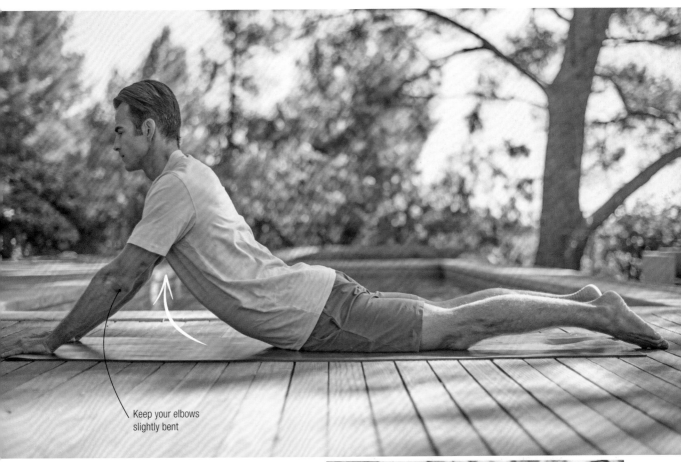

Keep your elbows
slightly bent

2 Press your palms into the ground to
lift your arms and chest off the ground,
broadening your chest and pulling your
shoulders back. **Hold.** Inhale and exhale
slow, steady breaths through your nose.
Slowly reverse out of the posture.

MAKE IT EASIER
In step 2, bend both knees as if you're going
to touch your toes to your head, but keep
your hips firmly planted on the ground.

Side seal

This asana is a variation of the classic Seal posture and helps to open up the side of the body in a restorative way. Side bends are a great way to boost your energy, and they help support healthy digestion, as well as improving your lateral spine flexibility.

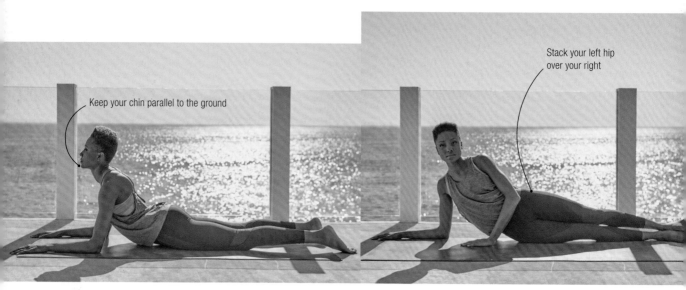

Keep your chin parallel to the ground

Stack your left hip over your right

1 Lie on your stomach and fully extend your legs behind you. Bend your elbows and keep your hands and forearms flat on the ground in front of you. Press your forearms into the ground to lift your chest and head off the ground.

2 Push on the ground with your left hand to roll onto your right hip and right forearm, keeping your legs extended and aligning your left leg on top of your right. Pull your shoulder blades back and lift your chest, placing your left hand flat on the ground in front of you for stability.

BE AWARE Place a folded blanket under your hips if you feel any discomfort there while holding the posture.

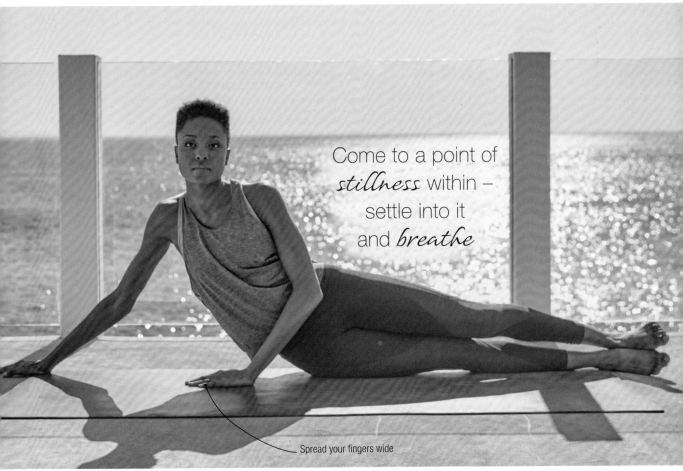

Come to a point of stillness within – settle into it and breathe

Spread your fingers wide

3 Press your right hand into the ground to straighten your right arm and extend your tailbone towards your heels. Pull the crown of your head upwards. **Hold.** Inhale and exhale slow, steady breaths through your nose. Slowly reverse out of the posture as you return to your starting position, then repeat on the opposite side.

MAKE IT EASIER
In step 2, bend your knees and place a block under the elbow of the extended arm for more support.

Banana

This beginner-friendly asana will give you a deep side stretch from your armpits to your legs, including your iliotibial (IT) band and obliques areas. Performing this in the morning can invigorate you for the entire day.

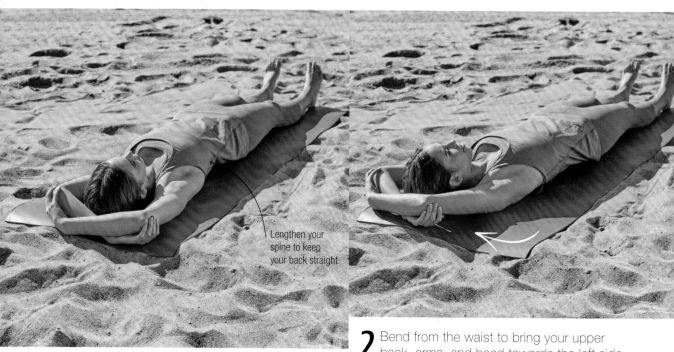

Lengthen your
spine to keep
your back straight

1 Lie on your back, extending your legs straight out in front of you. Reaching your arms over your head, grab your opposite elbows with your hands.

2 Bend from the waist to bring your upper back, arms, and head towards the left side of the mat, keeping your legs straight and your hips on the ground.

BE AWARE If you feel any discomfort in your arms or shoulders, keep your arms by your sides instead.

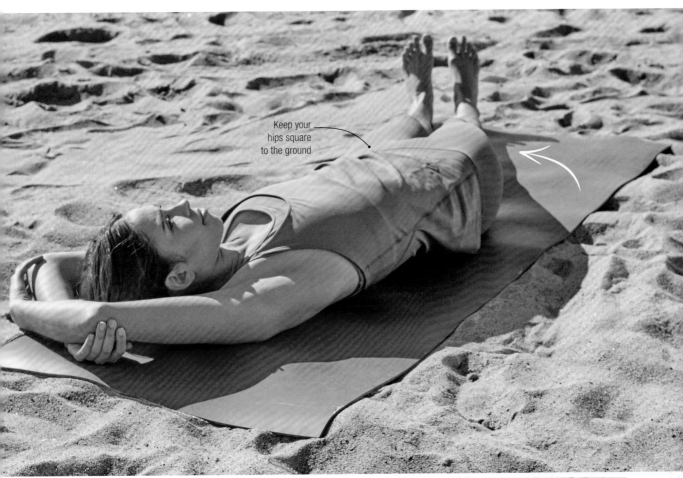

Keep your
hips square
to the ground

3 Complete the side bend by pressing your hips into the mat and walking your feet to the left until your body forms a banana shape. **Hold.** Inhale and exhale slow, steady breaths through your nose. Slowly reverse out of the posture as you return to your starting position, then repeat on the opposite side.

MAKE IT HARDER
In step 3, deepen the stretch in your IT band by crossing your right ankle over your left ankle, without lifting your right hip off the ground.

Straddle

This forward fold opens up your inner legs to improve lower-body flexibility while decompressing your spine. It is a great posture to do after a strong workout.

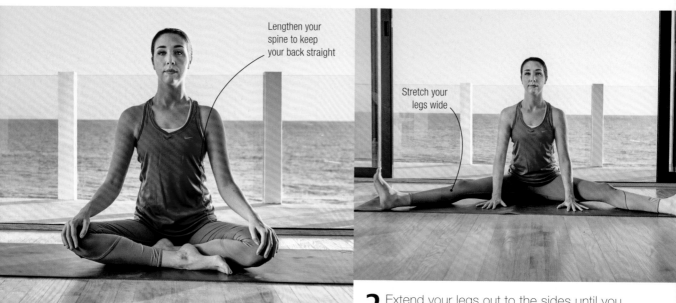

Lengthen your spine to keep your back straight

Stretch your legs wide

1 Sit on the ground in a comfortable position, crossing your legs and keeping your tailbone on the ground. Put your hands on your knees and extend the crown of your head upwards.

2 Extend your legs out to the sides until you find your edge. Put your hands flat on the ground in front of you, with your fingers pointing forwards, and keep your toes pointing straight up.

BE AWARE Although folding forwards could aggravate lower back injuries or sciatica, you can sit on a block or folded blankets to elevate your hips, or you can avoid folding forwards altogether.

Keep your back straight
and your spine aligned

3 Tilt your pelvis forwards
to initiate the forward fold,
and walk your hands out in front
of you for support.

Pull your shoulders
away from your ears

Settle into the
moment as you
focus on *breathing*

4 Once you find your edge, allow your spine to
round slightly. Allow gravity to pull you closer to the
ground. **Hold.** Inhale and exhale slow, steady breaths
through your nose. Slowly reverse out of the posture.

MAKE IT EASIER
In step 3, prop your hips up on
a block to help you tilt your pelvis
forwards, and place a block on its short
side under your forehead for support.

Dangling

This asana is the only one in this book you can do standing up, but it's a great way to lengthen your spine and stretch your hamstrings. Perform this forward fold to restore energy levels after a long day.

Keep your feet
hip-width apart

1 Stand tall, lengthening your spine, gently bending your knees, and relaxing your arms at your sides, with your palms facing forwards.

BE AWARE If you've suffered any kind of lower back injury, you can bend your knees more, or avoid this posture if you experience any pain.

Imagine *stress pouring out* from the top of your head with every exhale

Relax your neck

MAKE IT EASIER
In step 2, bend your knees even more to better support yourself during the fold.

2 Fold forwards at your hips, maintaining the gentle bend in your knees, and wrap your hands around the opposite elbows. Keep your weight evenly distributed through your feet, but allow gravity to take over. **Hold.** Inhale and exhale slow, steady breaths through your nose. Slowly reverse out of the posture.

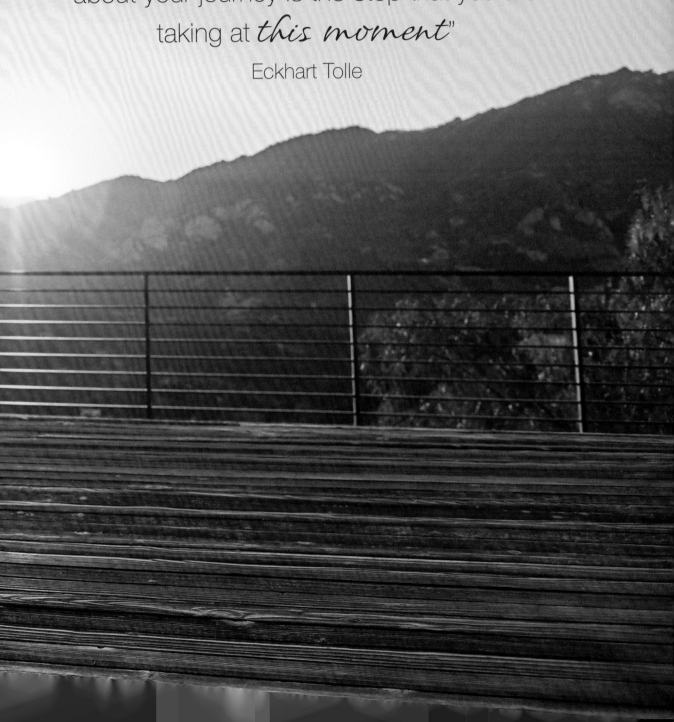

"The only thing that is *ultimately real* about your journey is the step that you are taking at *this moment*"

Eckhart Tolle

Snail

This intense asana provides the benefits of a forward fold combined with an inversion. It's a powerful way to stretch the back of your body – from the crown of your head, down your spine, and into your hamstrings.

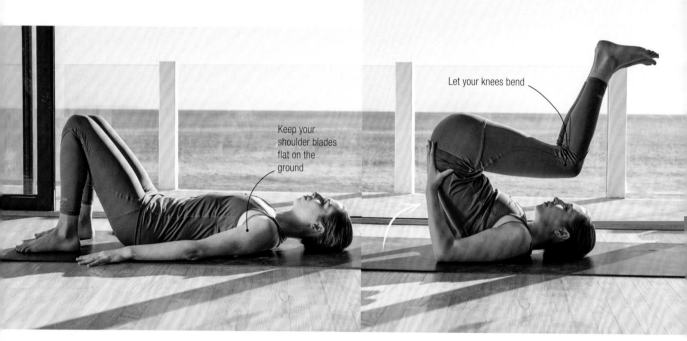

Keep your shoulder blades flat on the ground

Let your knees bend

1 Lie on your back and bend your knees, with your feet flat on the ground. Relax your arms at your sides and keep your hands flat on the ground.

2 Lift your hips and feet up so that your knees move towards your head, and place your hands behind your lower back. Let your spine and legs round to find your balance.

BE AWARE If you've ever experienced any kind of neck injury, or if you suffer from glaucoma, you should avoid this posture, since it can aggravate these conditions.

Keep your hips high

3 Straighten your legs back over your head so that your toes touch the ground behind you. Keep your hips elevated and straighten your arms out in front of you, with your palms facing up for stability. **Hold.** Inhale and exhale slow, steady breaths through your nose. Slowly reverse out of the posture.

MAKE IT HARDER
In step 3, bend your knees and rest them beside your ears, keeping your knees and the tops of your feet flat on the ground. Interlace your fingers, keeping your arms straight out in front of you and your elbows unbent.

Baby dragon

This asana does wonders for anyone who spends many hours sitting in a chair, and it can also prove therapeutic for sciatica. It stretches deeply into the front of your hips and creates length in your lower back.

Form a 90-degree angle with your right knee

1 Put your hands and knees on the ground, with your hands flat and your fingers pointing forwards. Keep your spine and neck parallel to the ground and your eyes looking down.

2 Step your right foot forwards, towards the top corner of your mat and positioned to the inside of your right hand, aligning your right knee directly over your right ankle.

BE AWARE If you have sensitive knees or have ever suffered any kind of knee injury, you might find this posture uncomfortable and should perform Knee to chest (page 84) instead.

Feel the pull of gravity a little more with each exhale

3 Extend your left leg behind you, allowing your hips to drop down. Keep your left knee on the ground and your arms straight, and lift your head to look forwards. Press down on your right big toe to keep your right foot flat on the ground, and let gravity pull your hips down. **Hold.** Inhale and exhale slow, steady breaths through your nose. Slowly reverse out of the posture as you return to your starting position, then repeat with the opposite leg.

MAKE IT EASIER
In step 3, place a block under each hand to keep your chest elevated.

Twisted dragon

This asana helps you stretch deeper into your legs by targeting your quadriceps. It also opens up the upper body and may provide some relief for lower back pain.

Always keep your right ankle under your knee

1 Put your hands and knees on the ground, with your hands flat and your fingers pointing forwards. Keep your spine and neck parallel to the ground and your eyes looking down.

2 Step your right foot forwards, towards the top corner of your mat and positioned to the inside of your right hand, aligning your right knee directly over your right ankle.

BE AWARE If you have sensitive knees or have suffered any kind of knee injury, you might find this posture uncomfortable and should perform the Lying quad stretch (page 58) instead.

Pull your shoulders
away from your ears

3 Extend your left leg behind you, allowing
your hips to drop down. Keep your left
knee on the ground.

4 Keep your left palm anchored to the ground
and extend your right arm towards the back
of the mat, twisting your upper body to the right.

MAKE IT EASIER
In step 5, use a strap
around the top of your
back foot.

5 Bend your left knee and grab the top of your left foot with your right
hand, pulling your left heel closer to your glutes. Soften your shoulders
and allow gravity to pull your hips down. **Hold.** Inhale and exhale slow,
steady breaths through your nose. Slowly reverse out of the posture as
you return to your starting position, then repeat with the opposite leg.

Dragon flying low

This asana goes deeper than the Baby dragon pose by applying more body weight to the hips. It's an intense hip-opening posture that deeply stretches your inner groin and hip flexors to increase mobility in the lower body.

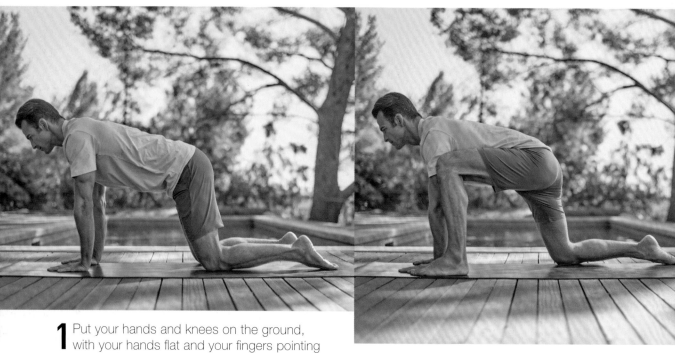

1 Put your hands and knees on the ground, with your hands flat and your fingers pointing forwards. Keep your spine and neck parallel to the ground and your eyes looking down.

2 Step your left foot forwards, towards the top corner of your mat and positioned to the outside of your left hand, aligning your left knee directly over your left ankle.

BE AWARE If you have sensitive knees or have ever suffered any kind of knee injury, place folded blankets under your knees.

3 Extend your right leg behind you, allowing your hips to drop down. Keep your right knee on the ground.

4 Slide your hands forwards to put your forearms flat on the ground. Allow your neck to relax so that your head hangs heavily. Press down on your left big toe to keep your left foot flat on the ground and let gravity pull your hips down. **Hold.** Inhale and exhale slow, steady breaths through your nose. Slowly reverse out of the posture as you return to your starting position, then repeat with the opposite leg.

MAKE IT EASIER
In step 4, place your forearms on two blocks or a bolster for support.

Winged dragon

This asana focuses on the outer rotation of your front hip to target the outer portion of your hip socket. It provides a very deep stretch for increased flexibility.

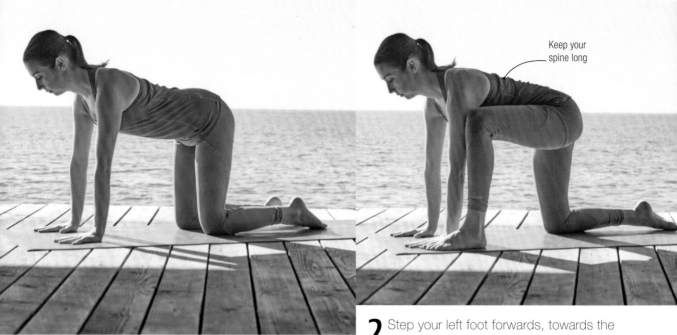

Keep your
spine long

1 Put your hands and knees on the ground, with your hands flat and your fingers pointing forwards. Keep your spine and neck parallel to the ground and your eyes looking down.

2 Step your left foot forwards, towards the top corner of your mat and positioned to the outside of your left hand, aligning your left knee directly over your left ankle.

BE AWARE If you have sensitive knees, ankles, or hips, or have ever suffered any kind of injury in these areas, perform the Sleeping swan (page 116) instead.

3 Extend your right leg behind you, allowing your hips to drop down. Keep your right knee on the ground as you lift your head to look forwards.

Internally repeat
"I am present"
with every exhale

Flex your right
foot to protect
your right knee

MAKE IT HARDER
In step 4, go deeper into your hip socket by sliding your hands forward so your forearms are flat on the ground. Let your eyes look down. You can place a block under your forehead or you can let your head hang heavily by relaxing your neck.

4 Rotate the front of your left hip outwards by rolling your left foot onto its outer side, and let gravity pull your left leg down. **Hold.** Inhale and exhale slow, steady breaths through your nose. Slowly reverse out of the posture as you return to your starting position, then repeat with the opposite leg.

Supported bridge

This simple asana offers an easy inversion – perfect for yin yoga beginners. It's a great pose to do if you suffer from lower back discomfort, or simply need to unwind after a long day. You'll need a block for this posture.

Form a straight line from your chest to your knees

Keep your shoulder blades flat on the ground

1 Lie on your back and bend your knees, keeping your feet flat on the ground. Relax your arms at your sides, with your left hand flat on the ground and a block under your right hand.

2 Press your feet into the ground to lift your hips off the ground, and use your core to help push through your feet.

BE AWARE If you have spine issues or have ever suffered any kind of spinal injury, use caution when doing backbends.

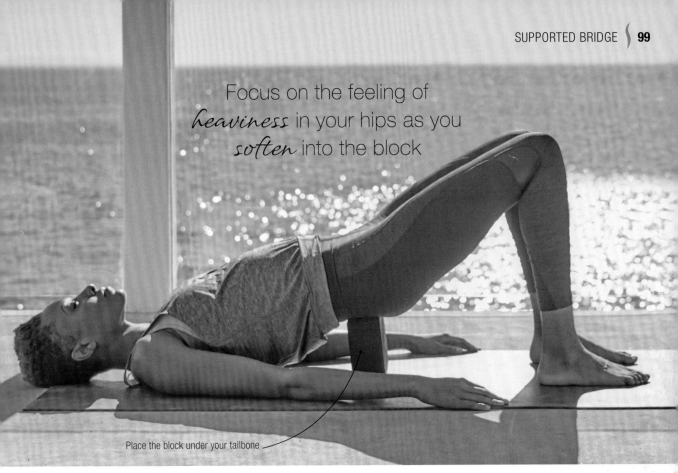

Focus on the feeling of
heaviness in your hips as you
soften into the block

Place the block under your tailbone

3 Position the block on its long side and place it directly under your hips. Rest your hips on the block and relax your arms by your sides. Keep your knees bent and your feet flat on the ground. **Hold.** Inhale and exhale slow, steady breaths through your nose. Slowly reverse out of the posture.

MAKE IT EASIER
In step 3, position your block flat on the ground under your hips.

MAKE IT HARDER
In step 3, position your block on the short side and straighten your legs out in front of you to stretch your hip flexors.

Pull your
shoulders back

1 Sit in a comfortable position, putting your hands on your knees. Keep your tailbone on the ground, cross your legs and extend the crown of your head upwards.

2 Reach your arms up in front of you and bend your elbows at 90-degree angles, aligning them with your shoulders. Face your palms towards each other.

Eagle arms

This upper-body asana broadens the space between your shoulder blades to enable deeper breathing. If you've got tight shoulders from working at a desk, or suffer from tension-induced headaches, you'll benefit from this posture.

BE AWARE If you've ever suffered any kind of rotator cuff injury, you should avoid this posture, especially if it causes you any pain.

3 Wrap your right arm under your left elbow and bring your right arm up until your forearms are parallel with your body.

Stay long through your spine

MAKE IT EASIER
In step 3, reach your hands to your opposite shoulders as though giving yourself a big hug. In step 4, hold this position.

4 Wrap your right wrist anticlockwise around your left wrist and place your palms together. Pull your shoulders down from your ears and push your elbows forwards. **Hold.** Inhale and exhale slow, steady breaths through your nose. Slowly reverse out of the posture as you return to your starting position, then switch arm positions and repeat.

Happy baby

This classic asana is a soothing way to target the muscles around your lower back while deeply opening up your hips and inner groin. It's an excellent posture to do first thing in the morning for an all-round stretch.

1 Lie on your back and bend your knees, with your feet flat on the ground. Relax your arms at your sides and keep your hands flat on the ground.

2 Bring your knees towards your chest and wrap your hands below your knees, opening them wide to bring them towards your shoulders and armpits. Press your tailbone into the ground to keep your spine level.

BE AWARE If you have a sensitive neck or have ever suffered any kind of neck injury, place a folded blanket or a block under your head for extra support.

Settle into *stillness* — focusing only on your breath as it *flows* through your nose

MAKE IT EASIER
In step 3, use a strap around each foot to pull your feet upwards.

3 Reach your arms up between your legs and grab your big toes with your fingers. Pull your feet up until the soles of your feet are facing upwards completely, keeping your knees bent. Pull your knees towards your chest without lifting your hips or head off the ground. **Hold.** Inhale and exhale slow, steady breaths through your nose. Slowly reverse out of the posture.

Thread the needle

This twisting asana focuses on the thoracic spine and is great preparation for doing backbends. It's also a calming posture that helps remove the kinks from your back after a night's sleep or a long day of standing on your feet.

1 Put your hands and knees on the ground, with your hands flat and your fingers pointing forwards. Keep your spine and neck parallel to the ground and your eyes looking down.

2 Reach your right arm underneath your body, rotate your upper body at your hips, and turn your head towards your left side.

BE AWARE If you've ever suffered any kind of neck or spine injury, use caution when practising twists, especially if you feel any pain.

Allow your back to gently twist to your right side

Breathe into your heart – feel it *expand* as you inhale and *soften* as you exhale

3 Bend your left elbow and lower your right shoulder and right ear to the ground.

MAKE IT EASIER
In steps 3 and 4, place your head on a block to provide support for your neck.

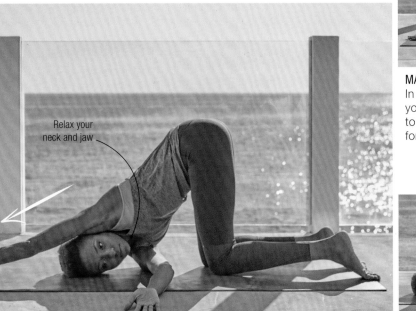

Relax your neck and jaw

4 Keep your hips aligned with your knees and extend your left arm forwards, keeping your elbow unbent and pressing your left palm into the ground to open up your upper back. **Hold.** Inhale and exhale slow, steady breaths through your nose. Slowly reverse out of the posture as you return to your starting position, then repeat with the opposite arm.

MAKE IT HARDER
In step 3, bend your left elbow and put your left hand behind your lower back.

"Remember, it doesn't
matter how *deep into a posture*
you go – what does matter is
who you are when you get there"

Max Strom

Bowtie

This asana provides a deep shoulder stretch using your own body weight to get into position. It's a calming pose that will help open up your upper back and can improve your posture by counteracting the rounding that occurs while sitting at a desk.

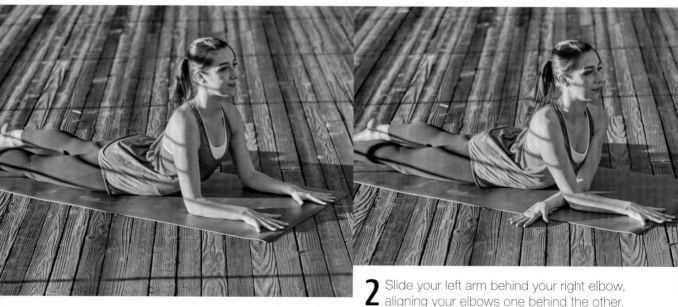

1 Lie on your stomach, with your legs fully extended behind you. Bend your elbows at 90-degree angles and place your hands flat on the ground in front of you. Lift your head and chest off the ground.

2 Slide your left arm behind your right elbow, aligning your elbows one behind the other. Turn your left palm upwards and press your forearms into the ground.

BE AWARE If you've ever suffered any kind of rotator cuff injury, you should avoid this posture, as it can aggravate the condition.

3 Turn your right arm so that it slides in the opposite direction to your left arm, continuing to align your elbows. Keep your right hand flat on the ground and continue to press your forearms into the ground.

Internally repeat *"I am"* as you inhale and *"at peace"* as you exhale

4 Extend your arms as far away from each other as you can. Lean forwards until your forehead touches the ground and your chest rests on top of your folded arms, letting gravity pull you down. **Hold.** Inhale and exhale slow, steady breaths through your nose. Slowly reverse out of the posture as you return to your starting position, then switch arm positions and repeat.

MAKE IT EASIER
In step 4, place a block or a bolster under your head to keep your chest elevated.

1 Sit in a comfortable position, crossing your legs and resting your hands on your knees. Keep your tailbone on the ground and extend the crown of your head upwards.

Press your hips down

2 Slide your left foot forward so your shin is roughly parallel to the top of your mat. (If you feel discomfort in your left knee, keep the heel of your left foot closer to your groin.)

Deer

This unique hip-opening asana combines inner and outer hip rotation to create balance in your hip joints. By adding a twist, this posture might also help stimulate digestion, relieve bloating, and soothe lower back discomfort.

BE AWARE If you have knee pain or have ever suffered any kind of knee injury, place a folded blanket under your front knee.

Keep your chest lifted and your shoulders back

3 Rotate your right foot out and extend your right leg behind you until your right shin is parallel with the side of the mat. Place your right hand on your left knee and your left hand flat on the ground for support.

Internally repeat *"I am enough"* as you hold this posture – let that statement *sink in*

4 Press down into your left hip to keep it close to the ground and lift up through your spine. Move into the twist by gently rotating your chest and shoulders towards your left side. **Hold.** Inhale and exhale slow, steady breaths through your nose. Slowly reverse out of the posture as you return to your starting position, then repeat with the opposite leg.

MAKE IT HARDER
In step 4, fold towards the side of your front leg. You can place a bolster under your chest for additional support.

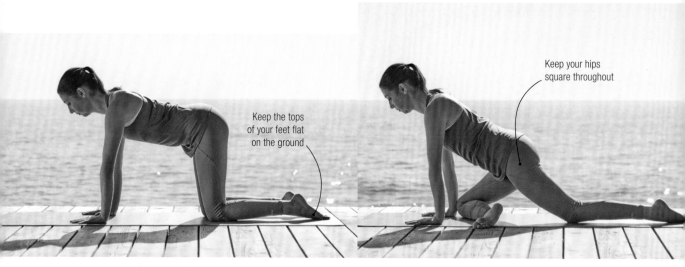

Keep the tops
of your feet flat
on the ground

Keep your hips
square throughout

1 Put your hands and knees on the ground, with your hands flat and your fingers pointing forwards. Keep your spine and neck parallel to the ground and your eyes looking down.

2 Slide your right foot forwards and underneath your body until your right knee reaches your right wrist, making your leg almost parallel with the top of the mat. Keep the outer side of your right foot flat on the ground.

Swan

This classic asana opens your hips through outer hip rotation – but it requires minimal effort to perform. This posture can also provide relief for lower body pain. Let gravity do most of the work for you, allowing your body to benefit even more.

BE AWARE If you have knee problems or limited hip mobility, perform the Seated swan (page 114) and Sleeping swan (page 116) instead.

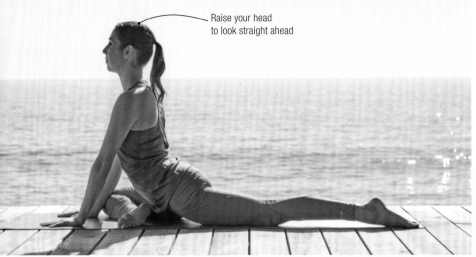

Raise your head
to look straight ahead

3 Fully extend your left leg behind you and lower
your hips to the ground, keeping the top of your
left foot flat on the ground.

MAKE IT EASIER
In step 3, place a block
flat on the ground under
your right hip. In step 4,
place a block on its short
side under your forehead.

Think about how *calm*
you begin to feel as you
breathe deeply

Keep your chest
lifted off the ground

4 Walk your hands forwards until your forearms and
elbows are flat on the ground. **Hold.** Inhale and exhale
slow, steady breaths through your nose. Slowly reverse out
of the posture as you return to your starting position, then
repeat with the opposite leg.

MAKE IT HARDER
In step 3, slide your
right leg to an even more
perpendicular position to
your body. In step 4, lean
forwards far enough to put
your head on the ground.

Seated swan

This asana promotes hip flexibility and takes a more cautious approach with your knees than the classic Swan, while still engaging the upper body. It can also relieve sciatica and can help improve your posture.

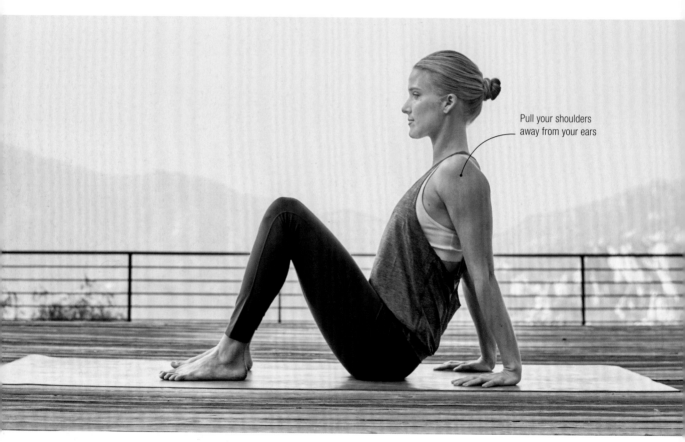

Pull your shoulders away from your ears

1 Sit on the ground, bend your knees and put your feet flat on the ground. Place your hands behind you for support, with your fingers pointing forwards.

BE AWARE If you've ever suffered lower back problems, use caution while performing this asana.

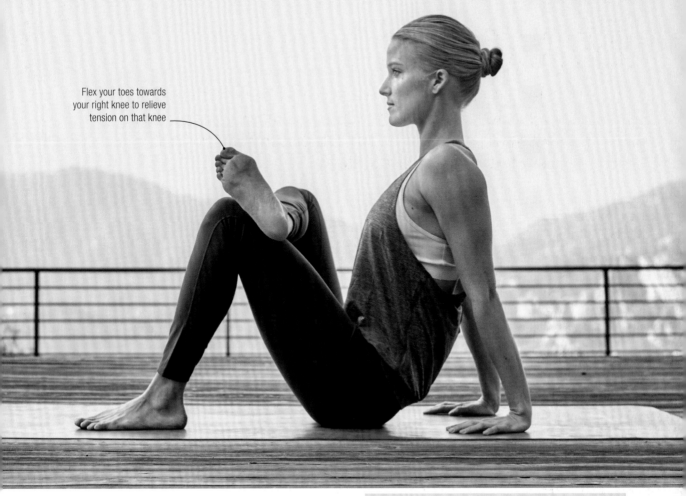

Flex your toes towards
your right knee to relieve
tension on that knee

2 Slowly bring your right foot over your left knee
and rest your right ankle just above your left
knee. Gently push your right knee away from your
body. **Hold.** Inhale and exhale slow, steady breaths
through your nose. Slowly reverse out of the
posture as you return to your starting position,
then repeat with the opposite leg.

MAKE IT EASIER
In step 2, place a bolster or block under
the foot that remains on the ground.

Sleeping swan

This is a more challenging version of the classic Swan asana. It will help you reach and improve the same muscles and tissues as that posture – including your hips, groin, glutes, and lower back – while reducing pressure on your knees.

Keep your shoulder blades and head flat on the ground

1 Lie on your back and bend your knees, with your feet flat on the ground. Relax your arms at your sides and keep your hands flat on the ground.

2 Slowly bring your right foot over your left knee and rest your right ankle just above your left knee. Flex your right toes towards your right knee to relieve tension on that knee, and gently push your right knee away from your body.

BE AWARE If you've ever suffered any neck or shoulder problems, use caution when performing this asana.

Internally say *"I am strong"* as you inhale
and *"I am stronger"* as you exhale

Continue to push your
knee away from your body

3 Reach your right arm through the opening
between your legs and reach your left arm
around the outside of your left leg. Intertwine your
fingers just below your left knee and pull your left
thigh towards your stomach. **Hold.** Inhale and
exhale slow, steady breaths through your nose.
Slowly reverse out of the posture as you return
to your starting position, then repeat with
the opposite leg.

MAKE IT EASIER
In step 1, place a bolster or a block
under your head.

Child's pose

In addition to stretching your back muscles, this classic asana calms your nerves and encourages the relaxation of body and mind. It's a wonderful posture to do when you need to unwind after a long day.

Keep your hands flat
and anchored to the ground

Keep your hips
aligned with
your ankles

1 Place your hands and knees on the ground, with your hands flat and your fingers pointing forwards. Keep your spine and neck parallel to the ground and your eyes looking down.

2 Bring your feet together until your big toes touch. Push your hips back and down, bringing them as close to your heels as possible, and rest your head on the ground.

BE AWARE If you have sensitive knees, you might find this posture uncomfortable and should perform the Reclined child's pose (page 120) instead.

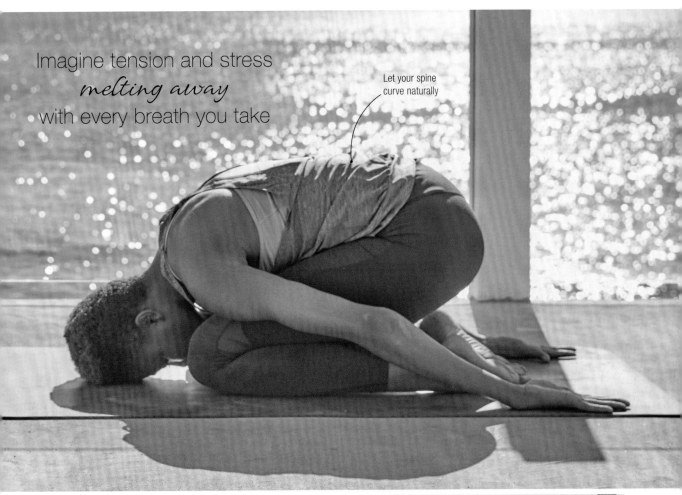

Imagine tension and stress
melting away
with every breath you take

Let your spine
curve naturally

3 Extend your arms towards the back of your mat,
turning your palms upwards and keeping the
backs of your hands flat on the ground. Let your
shoulders rest on your knees. **Hold.** Inhale and
exhale slow, steady breaths through your nose.
Slowly reverse out of the posture.

MAKE IT EASIER
In step 2, widen the space between your
knees and extend your arms further forward.

Reclined child's pose

This asana offers the same benefits as the traditional Child's pose, but it's easier on your knees. It's a restorative and meditative posture you can do anytime you feel stressed.

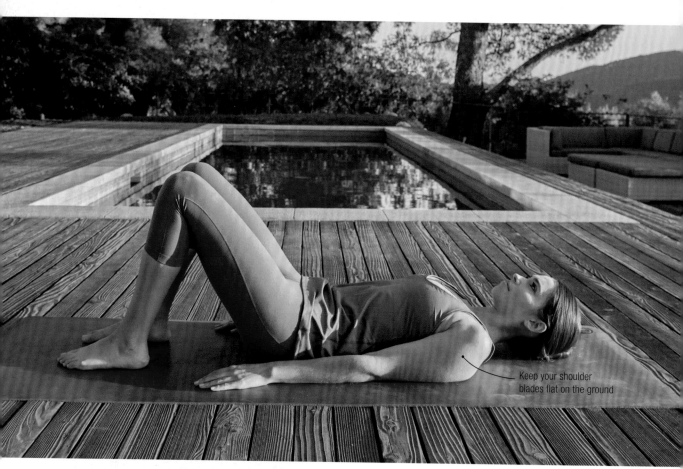

Keep your shoulder blades flat on the ground

1 Lie on your back and bend your knees, with your feet flat on the ground and your knees together. Relax your arms at your sides and keep your hands flat on the ground.

BE AWARE If lying flat on your back feels or becomes uncomfortable, place a pillow under your head to support your neck.

Pull your shoulders
away from your ears

2 Bring your knees towards your chest, wrap
your arms around your knees, and position
each hand just below its opposite knee. Keep
your head and shoulders on the ground, but lift
your tailbone off the ground. **Hold.** Inhale and
exhale slow, steady breaths through your nose.
Slowly reverse out of the posture.

When you *inhale*,
lengthen your spine, and when
you *exhale*, pull your
knees closer

MAKE IT HARDER
In step 2, widen your knees, place your hands
on your knees, and press your tailbone down.

Cat pulling its tail

This advanced asana combines a reclining twist with a slight backbend. It also stretches your iliotibial (IT) band and quadriceps to restore and revitalize the entire body, including relieving stiffness in your lower back.

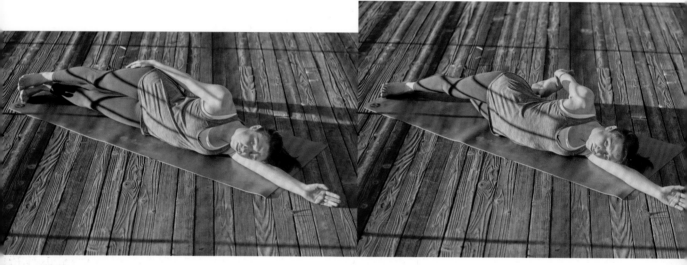

1 Lie on your left side, extending your left arm towards the top of your mat and placing your head on your arm. Place your right hand flat on the side of your right thigh and stack your right leg on top of your left leg.

2 Bend your left knee and reach your right arm behind you to grab the inside of your left foot with your right hand. Press your left heel out and away from your glutes, but keep your hips aligned.

BE AWARE If you have a sensitive lower back or have ever suffered any kind of lower back injury, you might want to avoid this posture.

3 Slide your right leg out towards the left side of your mat until it's parallel with the bottom of your mat. Reach your left hand out to grab your right big toe. Keep your head flat on the ground.

MAKE IT EASIER
In step 3, prop yourself on your left forearm and let your right leg go out to the side on its own. Keep holding your left foot with your right hand. In step 4, hold this position.

4 Move into a spinal twist by dropping your right shoulder towards the ground and keeping your right hip stacked over your left hip as much as possible. **Hold.** Inhale and exhale slow, steady breaths through your nose. Slowly reverse out of the posture as you return to your starting position, then repeat with the opposite leg.

Supported fish

This restorative asana connects with your heart chakra and helps balance your energy levels. It also invites you to breathe deeply into your chest and stretches the muscles around your ribcage. You'll need two blocks for this posture.

Keep your hips on the ground

1 Place two blocks on their long sides behind you, one placed lengthways for your upper back and one widthways for your head. Sit on the ground, bending your knees and keeping your feet flat on the ground, with your hands behind you and your fingers pointing forwards.

2 Use your arms to gently lie yourself back on the blocks – adjusting them as needed – so that your upper back, neck, and head are supported. Position your arms at your sides, with your hands flat on the ground and your palms facing up.

BE AWARE If you've ever suffered any kind of back injury, use caution when doing backbends. Go slowly – and stop if you experience any pain.

Internally repeat the affirmation
"I am open and receptive to love"

Close your eyes –
and relax

3 Extend your legs out in front of you to allow your hips and lower back to settle into the ground. **Hold.** Inhale and exhale slow, steady breaths through your nose. Slowly reverse out of the posture.

MAKE IT HARDER
In step 3, reach your arms over your head, touching the ground with the backs of your fingers. Push your bent knees outwards to bring the soles of your feet together.

"Change yourself – *you are in control*"

Mahatma Gandhi

Melting heart

As its name suggests, this asana opens up the area near your heart by stretching deeply into your shoulders and the muscles around your ribcage. It can also help soothe and relax your nerves.

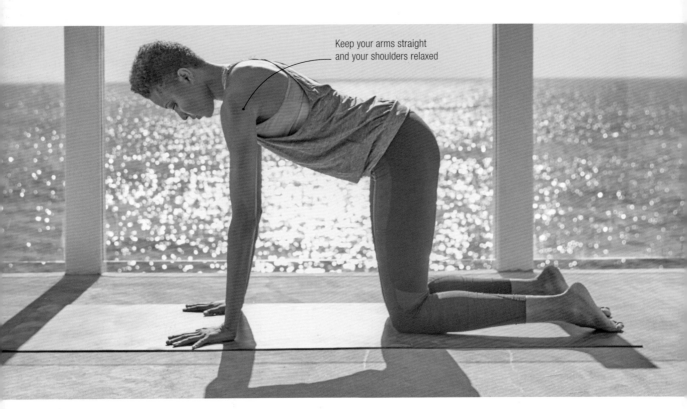

Keep your arms straight and your shoulders relaxed

1 Put your hands and knees on the ground, with your hands flat and your fingers pointing forwards. Keep your spine and neck parallel to the ground and your eyes looking down.

BE AWARE If you have sensitive knees, place a folded blanket underneath them. If you've suffered any kind of neck injury, you might find this posture uncomfortable.

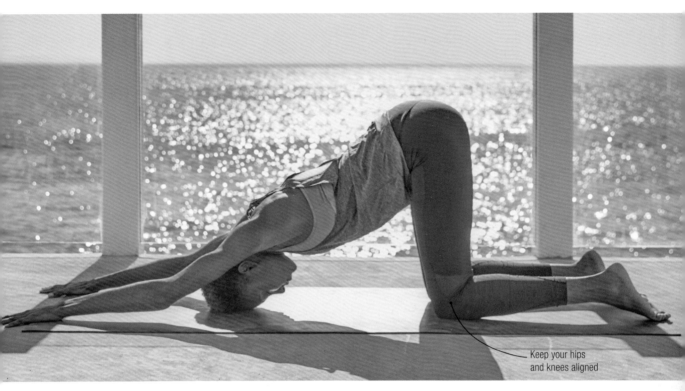

Keep your hips
and knees aligned

2 Walk your hands out in front of you until you can lower
your forehead to the ground. Reach through your arms,
soften your neck and upper back, and feel your ribcage
expand. **Hold.** Inhale and exhale slow, steady breaths
through your nose. Slowly reverse out of the posture.

MAKE IT EASIER
In step 2, if your forehead doesn't touch the
ground, place a block underneath it for support.

MAKE IT HARDER
In step 2, place one block under each elbow
to elevate your arms. Press your hands together
and bend your elbows so that your hands rest
on the back of your head. This allows you to go
deeper into the posture to stretch your triceps.

Legs up the wall

This beginner-friendly asana is the perfect posture to do after a long day of standing on your feet or following a vigorous workout. This mild inversion will help soothe and restore aching legs and prepare you for deep sleep.

1 Sit in a comfortable position 15cm (6in) away from a wall, with your right side towards the wall and your hands on your knees. Keep your tailbone on the ground, cross your legs, and extend the crown of your head upwards.

2 Lie gently on your back, rotating your body until your tailbone faces the wall. Rest the bottom of your feet flat on the wall and bend your knees towards your stomach. Relax your head and neck.

BE AWARE Because inversions can increase the pressure around your eyes, this posture isn't suitable for anyone suffering from glaucoma.

Think *"I am"*
as you inhale
and *"at ease"*
as you exhale

MAKE IT HARDER
In step 3, bring your hips
closer to the wall and widen
your legs as far as possible.

3 Fully extend your legs upwards to rest your heels against
the wall, keeping a slight bend in your knees to avoid
hyperextending them. **Hold.** Inhale and exhale slow, steady
breaths through your nose. Slowly reverse out of the posture.

Stack one
knee over
the other

1 Sit in a comfortable position, with your
hands on your knees. Keep your tailbone
on the ground, cross your legs and extend
the crown of your head upwards.

2 Slide your left foot to your right side
and your right foot to your left side until
your knees are aligned. Pull your feet
towards your hips and place your hands
flat on the ground behind you for support.

Shoelace

This seated asana combines the benefits of hip-openers and
forward folds to help you decompress and unwind when you're
feeling stressed or distraught. It can also help relieve lower back
pain and soothe your nervous system.

BE AWARE If you have limited hip flexibility, perform
the Reclined shoelace (page 134) instead.

3 Walk your hands out in front of you, slightly bending your elbows, to initiate the forward fold.

If your *mind* wanders, bring your *awareness* back to your breath

4 Straighten your arms, spread your fingers wide, and fold forwards until you find your edge, keeping your tailbone anchored to the ground. **Hold.** Inhale and exhale slow, steady breaths through your nose. Slowly reverse out of the posture as you return to your starting position, then repeat with opposite leg positions.

MAKE IT EASIER
In step 2, place a folded blanket or a block between your knees for extra support. In step 4, you can also place a bolster under your chest.

Reclined shoelace

This milder version of the Shoelace asana targets the outer hips without placing too much pressure on your joints. It might also offer relief if you suffer from sciatica.

Lengthen your spine

1 Lie on your back and bend your knees, with your feet flat on the ground. Relax your arms at your sides and keep your hands flat on the ground.

2 Lift your legs off the ground and cross your right calf over your left knee, aligning your knees as much as possible. Lightly flex your feet towards your knees.

BE AWARE If you've ever suffered any kind of knee injury, you might find this uncomfortable. When practising this asana, keep your feet flexed to maintain integrity in your knee joints.

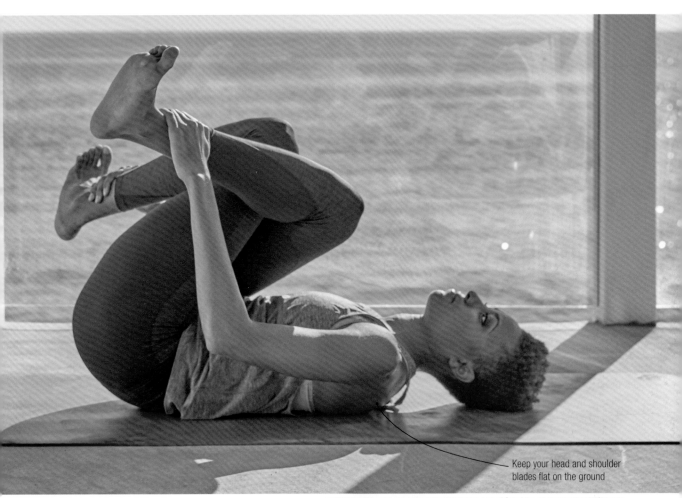

Keep your head and shoulder blades flat on the ground

3 Grasp your ankles with your hands and bend your elbows to pull your legs closer to your stomach. **Hold.** Inhale and exhale slow, steady breaths through your nose. Slowly reverse out of the posture as you return to your starting position, then repeat with the opposite leg.

MAKE IT EASIER
In step 3, wrap a strap around your shins.

Reverse prayer arms

This upper body asana is a great way to stretch your wrists and relieve aches and pains after working at a computer. It also opens up your chest and shoulders, helping to promote good posture.

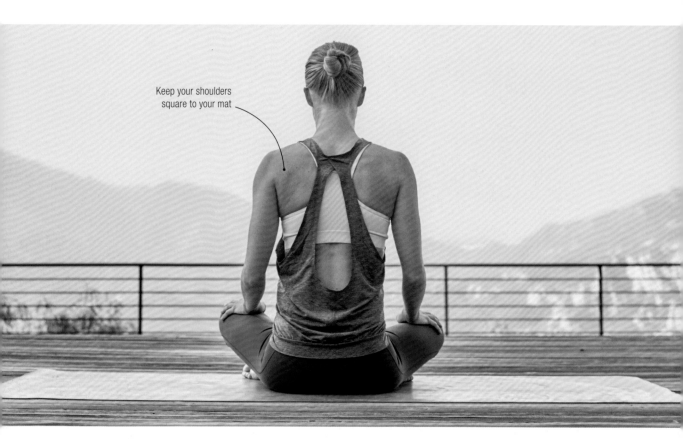

Keep your shoulders square to your mat

1 Sit in a comfortable position, with your hands on your knees. Keep your tailbone on the ground, cross your legs, and extend the crown of your head upwards.

BE AWARE If you've ever suffered any kind of rotator cuff or wrist injury, you might want to avoid this posture, especially if it causes pain.

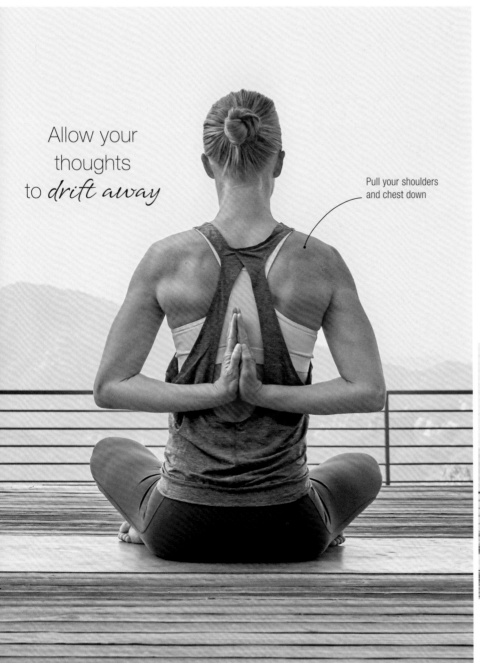

Allow your
thoughts
to *drift away*

Pull your shoulders
and chest down

MAKE IT EASIER
In step 2, wrap your hands
around your wrists.

2 Reach your arms behind your back, bending your elbows, and press your palms and fingers together, with your fingertips pointing up. **Hold.** Inhale and exhale slow, steady breaths through your nose. Slowly reverse out of the posture.

Frog

This simple yet intense asana will help you open up your inner thighs and groin to improve hip flexibility. You'll need two blankets for this posture.

Flex your feet
to protect your knees

1 Place a folded blanket on either side of your mat. Place your hands and knees on the ground, with your hands flat and fingers pointing forwards. Keep your spine and neck parallel to the ground and your eyes looking down.

2 Widen your knees as far as comfortable, making sure they stay aligned with your hips, and place them on the blankets. Align your ankles with your knees and flex your feet so that your toes point out to the sides.

BE AWARE If you have tight hips or sensitive knees and ankles, you might find this posture uncomfortable, so use a bolster for added support or perform the Child's pose (page 118) instead.

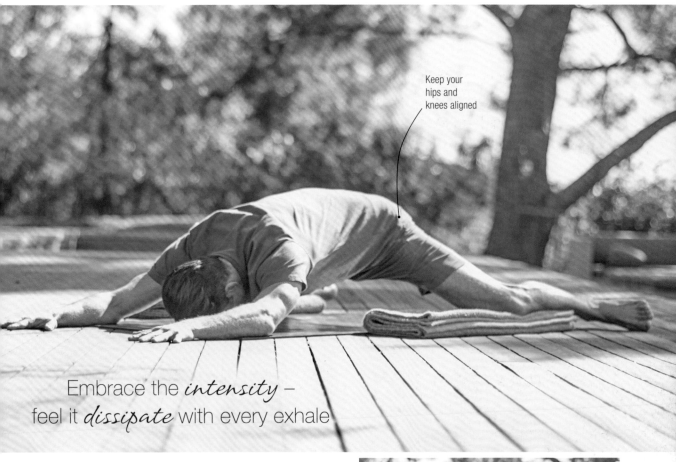

Keep your
hips and
knees aligned

*Embrace the intensity –
feel it dissipate with every exhale*

3 Without changing the alignment of your lower body, keep your chest lifted as you bend your elbows and walk your hands forwards until your forearms, elbows, and forehead touch the ground. Allow gravity to pull your hips down. **Hold.** Inhale and exhale slow, steady breaths through your nose. Slowly reverse out of the posture.

MAKE IT EASIER
In step 3, place a bolster or two under your upper body and head, and angle your legs to allow you to touch your big toes together.

Half monkey

This asana opens up your hamstrings and prepares you for the full Monkey posture. Runners especially will benefit from this asana, because it stretches the hamstrings, groin, and calves.

Lengthen your spine

1 Put your hands and knees on the ground, with your hands flat and your fingers pointing forwards. Keep your spine and neck parallel to the ground and your eyes looking down.

2 Step your right foot forwards, towards the top corner of your mat and positioned to the inside of your right hand, aligning your right knee directly over your right ankle.

BE AWARE If you've ever suffered any kind of groin or hamstring tear, use caution during this posture, since it could aggravate either condition.

3 Straighten your right leg and shift your hips back until they align over your left knee. Walk your hands forwards on your fingertips until your fingers align with your right ankle. Keep the top of your left foot flat on the ground and your right leg supported on the heel of your right foot.

Let your upper back round

MAKE IT EASIER
In step 3, place a block under each palm and keep your chest elevated. You can also slightly bend your front knee.

4 Place your hands flat on the ground and fold forwards towards your right knee. **Hold.** Inhale and exhale slow, steady breaths through your nose. Slowly reverse out of the posture as you return to your starting position, then repeat with the opposite leg.

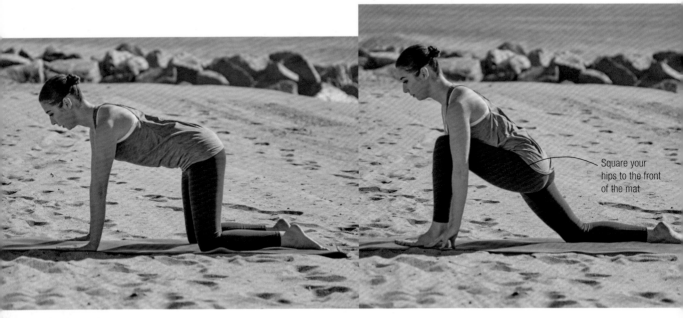

Square your
hips to the front
of the mat

1 Put your hands and knees on the ground, with your hands flat and your fingers pointing forwards. Keep your spine and neck parallel to the ground and your eyes looking down.

2 Step your left foot forwards, towards the top corner of your mat and positioned to the inside of your left hand, aligning your left knee directly over your left ankle. Align your hands with your left ankle and use your fingertips for balance.

Monkey

This advanced asana is a deep hip opener, as well as an intense hamstring stretch. The key is to go into this posture slowly and mindfully, never rushing the process.

BE AWARE If you've ever suffered any kind of groin injury or hamstring tear, use caution, since this posture could aggravate either condition.

Keep your head
and spine aligned

3 Extend your left foot
forwards as far as
you can and shift your
hips back until they align
over your right knee.

Soften
your arms

4 Extend your right leg behind you, letting
gravity pull your hips down as you put your
hands flat on the ground for support. **Hold.**
Inhale and exhale slow, steady breaths through
your nose. Slowly reverse out of the posture
as you return to your starting position, then
switch leg positions and repeat.

MAKE IT EASIER
In step 4, place a block or a bolster
under your hips.

Corpse

This classic asana is the last posture performed during any yin yoga practice. It helps rejuvenate your mind and body, and is a vital component in any yin yoga sequence.

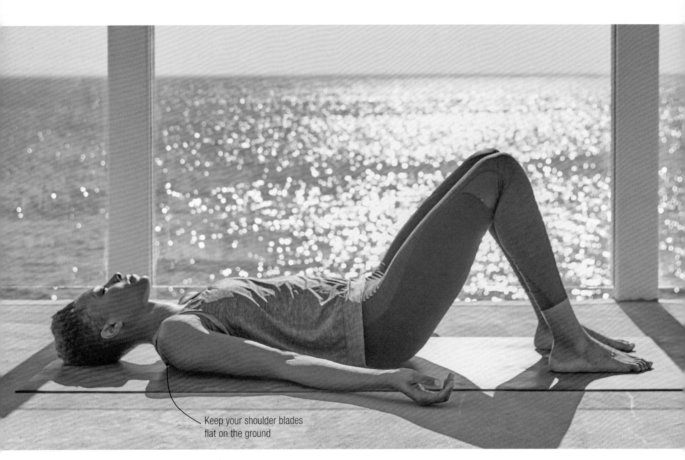

Keep your shoulder blades flat on the ground

1 Lie on your back and bend your knees, keeping your feet flat on the ground. Relax your arms at your sides, with your fingers curled slightly upwards.

As you inhale, picture a *wave of peace* washing over you, and as you exhale, picture the *wave taking away stress*

Allow your inner ankles to roll outwards

2 Extend your legs out one at a time, placing your heels towards the sides of the mat and letting gravity pull your feet down. Pull your shoulders down from your ears and extend your hands. **Hold.** Inhale and exhale slow, steady breaths through your nose. Slowly reverse out of the posture.

MAKE IT EASIER
In step 2, place a block under each knee.

Yin sequences

Within this chapter you'll practise sequences that combine asanas into unique flows, helping you reach a variety of goals. Ranging from 30 minutes to 90 minutes, these sequences are perfect for yoga beginners and veterans.

TOTAL TIME »

60
minutes

Pre-workout stretch

This is excellent to do before exercises that actively engage your muscles and elevate your heart rate. It is also a good sequence for days between workouts to help your joints heal and recover.

REQUIRED PROP
• 1 blanket

OPTIONAL PROPS
• 2 blocks
• 1 bolster
• 1 strap

START

SEATED MEDITATION	TOE SQUAT	ANKLE STRETCH	HALF MONKEY
page 24	page 38	page 44	page 140
hold for **5 mins**	hold for **3 mins**	hold for **3 mins**	hold for **4 mins** on each side

Beginner sequence

This hour-long practice is a great intro to yin yoga if you're new to it. The reclined postures for these asanas also make this sequence ideal if you have a limited range of motion in your hips and lower back.

REQUIRED PROP
- 1 strap

OPTIONAL PROPS
- 2 blocks

START

SEATED MEDITATION page 24	**HUMMING BEE BREATH** page 19	**CHILD'S POSE** page 118	**LYING QUAD STRETCH** page 58
hold for **6 mins**	perform for **5 mins**	hold for **5 mins**	hold for **3 mins** on each side

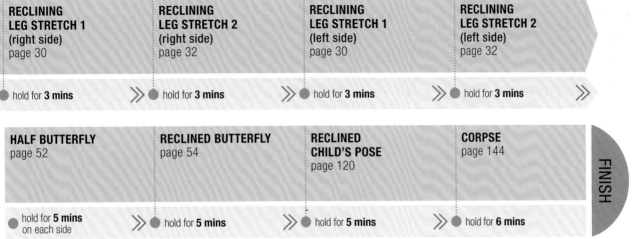

RECLINING LEG STRETCH 1 (right side) page 30	RECLINING LEG STRETCH 2 (right side) page 32	RECLINING LEG STRETCH 1 (left side) page 30	RECLINING LEG STRETCH 2 (left side) page 32	
hold for **3 mins**	hold for **3 mins**	hold for **3 mins**	hold for **3 mins**	

HALF BUTTERFLY page 52	RECLINED BUTTERFLY page 54	RECLINED CHILD'S POSE page 120	CORPSE page 144	FINISH
hold for **5 mins** on each side	hold for **5 mins**	hold for **5 mins**	hold for **6 mins**	

TOTAL TIME »

60
minutes

Improving your digestion

This sequence might provide relief if you're suffering from digestive issues. As you twist and fold forwards while performing these asanas, you compress and decompress your stomach, helping to stimulate healthy digestion.

REQUIRED PROPS
• none

OPTIONAL PROPS
• block
• bolster
• strap

SEATED MEDITATION page 24	ALTERNATE NOSTRIL BREATH page 18	SQUAT page 36	CATERPILLAR page 48	SQUARE page 28
hold for **6 mins**	perform for **5 mins**	hold for **3 mins**	hold for **5 mins**	hold for **5 mins** on each side

RECLINED CHILD'S POSE
page 120

hold for **5 mins**

RECLINED SHOELACE
page 134

hold for **5 mins** on each side

LYING SPINAL TWIST
page 60

hold for **5 mins** on each side

CORPSE
page 144

hold for **6 mins**

FINISH

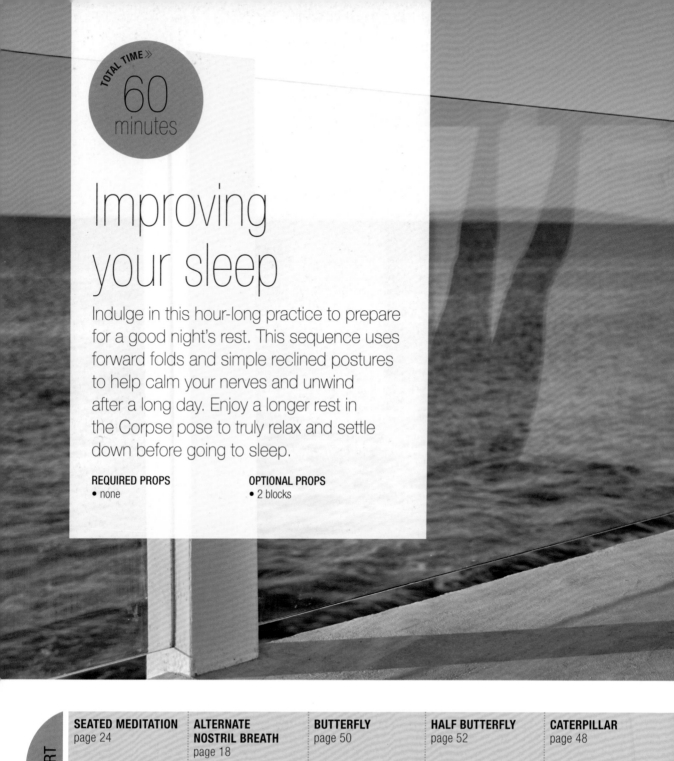

60 minutes

Improving your sleep

Indulge in this hour-long practice to prepare for a good night's rest. This sequence uses forward folds and simple reclined postures to help calm your nerves and unwind after a long day. Enjoy a longer rest in the Corpse pose to truly relax and settle down before going to sleep.

REQUIRED PROPS
• none

OPTIONAL PROPS
• 2 blocks

START

SEATED MEDITATION page 24	**ALTERNATE NOSTRIL BREATH** page 18	**BUTTERFLY** page 50	**HALF BUTTERFLY** page 52	**CATERPILLAR** page 48
hold for **5 mins**	perform for **5 mins**	hold for **5 mins**	hold for **5 mins** on each side	hold for **5 mins**

FINISH

hold for **5 mins**
on each side   ≫   hold for **5 mins**   ≫   hold for **5 mins**   ≫   hold for **10 mins**

Improving your energy

This short sequence will provide you with a natural boost of energy when you feel drained or fatigued. It's great to perform when you wake up in the morning or when you need to get focused and energized later in the day.

REQUIRED PROPS
• none

OPTIONAL PROPS
• 1 strap
• 1 block

START

SEATED MEDITATION	DANGLING	DEER	SIDE SEAL
page 24	page 84	page 110	page 78
hold for **3 mins**	hold for **3 mins**	hold for **3 mins** on each side	hold for **3 mins** on each side

CAT PULLING ITS TAIL page 122	SNAIL page 88	CORPSE page 144	FINISH
hold for **3 mins** on each side	hold for **3 mins**	hold for **3 mins**	

TOTAL TIME »

60
minutes

Intermediate sequence

This hour-long sequence is perfect if you want an overall stretch and already have some flexibility in your hips, hamstrings, and lower back. Focus on the flow of your breath and the tension releasing from your joints as you hold the postures.

REQUIRED PROP
• 1 strap

OPTIONAL PROPS
• 1 additional strap
• 2 blocks

START

SEATED MEDITATION page 24	ALTERNATE NOSTRIL BREATH page 18	REVERSE PRAYER ARMS with TOE SQUAT pages 136 and 38	WINGED DRAGON page 96
● hold for **5 mins**	● perform for **5 mins**	● hold for **5 mins**	● hold for **5 mins** on each side

STRADDLE page 82	**RECLINED SHOELACE** page 134	**HAPPY BABY** page 102	**RECLINING LEG STRETCH 1** (right side) page 30
hold for **5 mins**	hold for **5 mins** on each side	hold for **3 mins**	hold for **3 mins**

CAT PULLING ITS TAIL (right side) page 122	**RECLINING LEG STRETCH 1** (left side) page 30	**CAT PULLING ITS TAIL** (left side) page 122	**CORPSE** page 144	FINISH
hold for **3 mins**	hold for **3 mins**	hold for **3 mins**	hold for **5 mins**	

Neck & shoulder tension relief

This short sequence focuses on your neck and shoulders, helping to eliminate kinks in your upper body. It can also support the healthy flow of energy through your heart and lung meridians, and your throat chakra.

REQUIRED PROPS
• none

OPTIONAL PROPS
• 1 strap
• 1 block

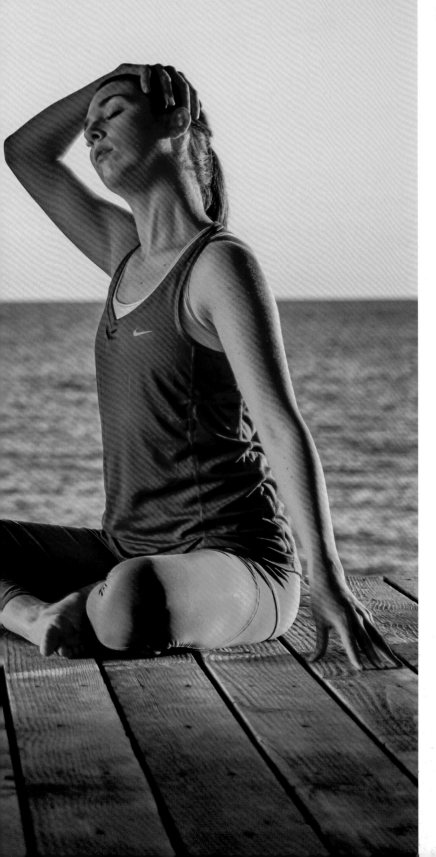

START

SEATED MEDITATION
page 24

hold for **3 mins**

⌄⌄

NECK RELEASE
page 42

hold for **3 mins**
on each side

⌄⌄

BOWTIE
page 108

hold for **3 mins**
on each side

⌄⌄

ARCHER ARMS
page 64

hold for **3 mins**
on each side

⌄⌄

LYING CHEST OPENER
page 56

hold for **3 mins**
on each side

⌄⌄

CORPSE
page 144

hold for **3 mins**

FINISH

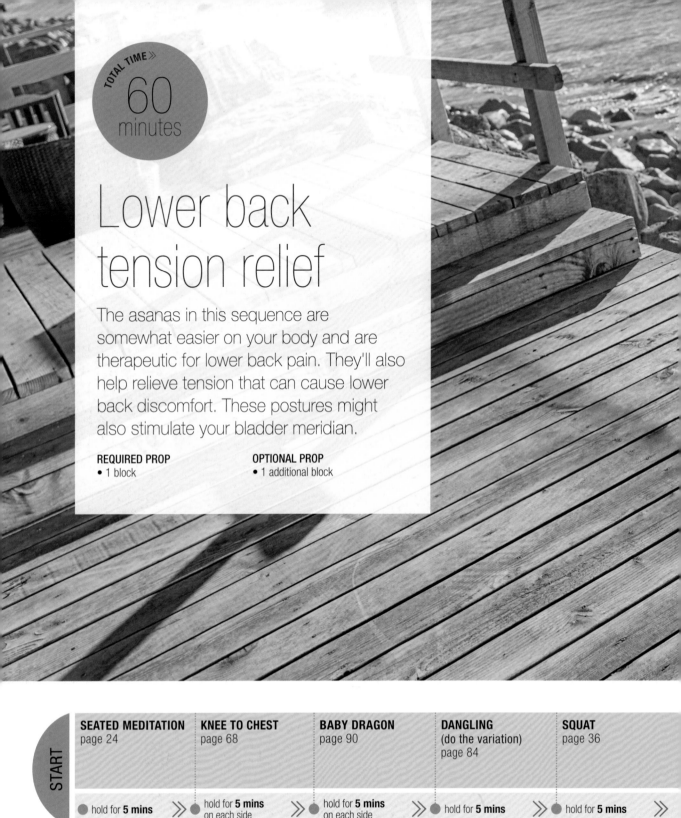

TOTAL TIME ≫

60
minutes

Lower back tension relief

The asanas in this sequence are somewhat easier on your body and are therapeutic for lower back pain. They'll also help relieve tension that can cause lower back discomfort. These postures might also stimulate your bladder meridian.

REQUIRED PROP
• 1 block

OPTIONAL PROP
• 1 additional block

START	SEATED MEDITATION page 24	KNEE TO CHEST page 68	BABY DRAGON page 90	DANGLING (do the variation) page 84	SQUAT page 36
	● hold for **5 mins** ≫	● hold for **5 mins** on each side ≫	● hold for **5 mins** on each side ≫	● hold for **5 mins** ≫	● hold for **5 mins** ≫

**RECLINED
CHILD'S POSE**
page 120

SUPPORTED BRIDGE
page 98

LYING SPINAL TWIST
page 60

CORPSE
(do the variation)
page 144

FINISH

hold for **5 mins**

hold for **5 mins**

hold for **5 mins**
on each side

hold for **5 mins**

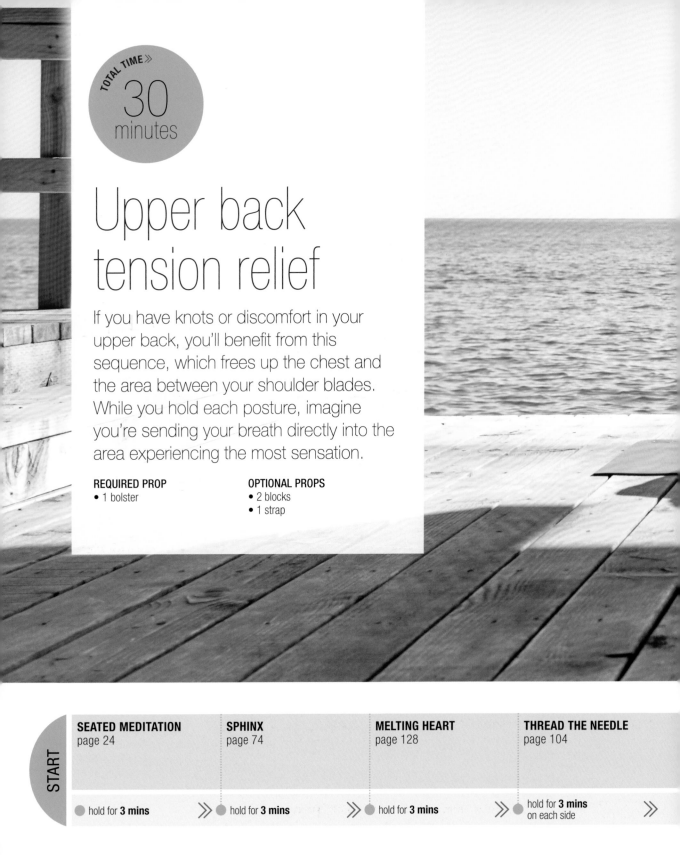

TOTAL TIME »

30 minutes

Upper back tension relief

If you have knots or discomfort in your upper back, you'll benefit from this sequence, which frees up the chest and the area between your shoulder blades. While you hold each posture, imagine you're sending your breath directly into the area experiencing the most sensation.

REQUIRED PROP
• 1 bolster

OPTIONAL PROPS
• 2 blocks
• 1 strap

START

SEATED MEDITATION page 24	SPHINX page 74	MELTING HEART page 128	THREAD THE NEEDLE page 104
hold for **3 mins**	hold for **3 mins**	hold for **3 mins**	hold for **3 mins** on each side

EAGLE ARMS
page 100

SUPPORTED FISH
page 124

CORPSE
page 144

FINISH

hold for **3 mins**
on each side

〉〉 hold for **3 mins**

〉〉 hold for **6 mins**

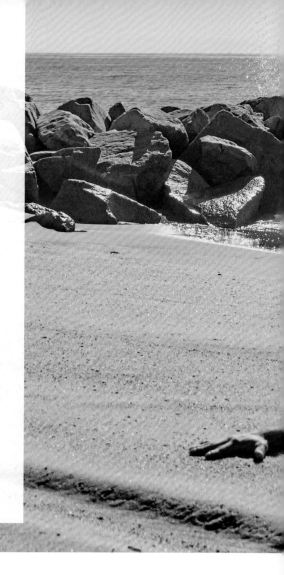

90 minutes

Advanced sequence

This sequence takes you through some more advanced asanas that will deeply stretch your spine, hips, and hamstrings. It's for more experienced yoga practitioners who already have good flexibility.

REQUIRED PROPS
• none

OPTIONAL PROPS
• 1 strap
• 2 blocks
• 1 bolster

START

SEATED MEDITATION page 24	**CATERPILLAR** page 48	**SHOELACE with ARCHER ARMS** pages 132 and 64	**STRADDLE** page 82
hold for **5 mins**	hold for **10 mins**	hold for **5 mins** on each side	hold for **10 mins**

FROG
page 138

hold for **5 mins**

SWAN
page 112

hold for **5 mins**
on each side

TWISTED DRAGON
page 92

hold for **5 mins**
on each side

SADDLE
page 62

hold for **5 mins**

SNAIL
page 88

hold for **5 mins**

LYING SPINAL TWIST
page 60

hold for **5 mins**
on each side

CORPSE
page 144

hold for **10 mins**

FINISH

TOTAL TIME »

90
minutes

Relieving stress

The gentle asanas in this meditative sequence will help you unwind after a stressful day so you can clear your thoughts and focus on the present moment. Imagine tension melting away from your mind and body with each exhale.

REQUIRED PROPS
• none

OPTIONAL PROPS
• 1 block
• 2 straps

START

SEATED MEDITATION page 24	**ALTERNATE NOSTRIL BREATH** page 18	**RECLINED CHILD'S POSE** page 120	**KNEE TO CHEST** page 68
● hold for **5 mins**	● perform for **5 mins**	● hold for **5 mins**	● hold for **5 mins** on each side

MELTING HEART
page 128

● hold for **5 mins**

HAPPY BABY
page 102

hold for **5 mins**

IT BAND STRETCH
page 40

hold for **5 mins**
on each side

DANGLING
page 84

hold for **5 mins**

SQUAT
page 36

hold for **5 mins**

THREAD THE NEEDLE
page 104

hold for **5 mins**
on each side

CATERPILLAR
page 48

hold for **5 mins**

LYING SPINAL TWIST
page 60

hold for **5 mins**
on each side

CORPSE
page 144

hold for **10 mins**

FINISH

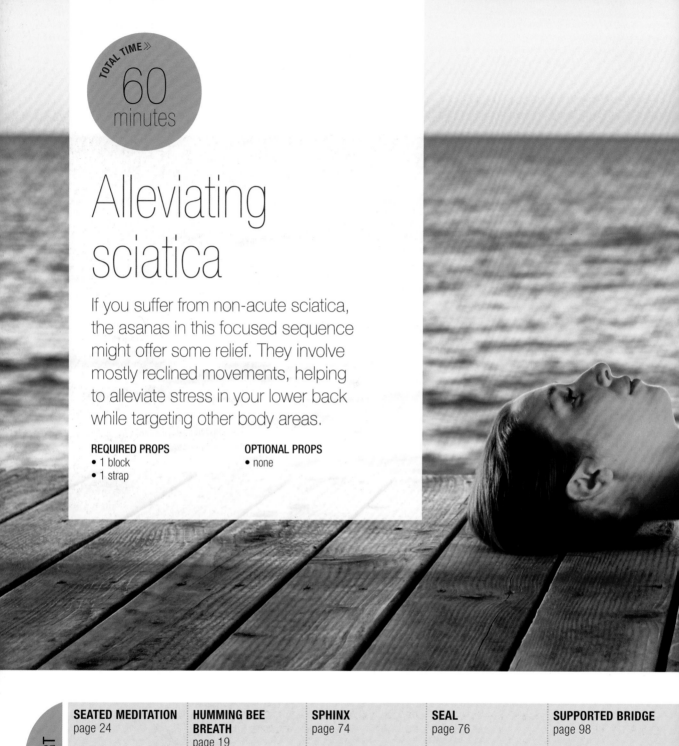

Alleviating sciatica

If you suffer from non-acute sciatica, the asanas in this focused sequence might offer some relief. They involve mostly reclined movements, helping to alleviate stress in your lower back while targeting other body areas.

REQUIRED PROPS
• 1 block
• 1 strap

OPTIONAL PROPS
• none

START

SEATED MEDITATION page 24	HUMMING BEE BREATH page 19	SPHINX page 74	SEAL page 76	SUPPORTED BRIDGE page 98
hold for **5 mins**	perform for **5 mins**	hold for **5 mins**	hold for **5 mins**	hold for **5 mins**

**RECLINING
LEG STRETCH 1**
page 30

SLEEPING SWAN
page 116

RECLINED SHOELACE
page 134

CORPSE
page 144

FINISH

hold for **5 mins**
on each side

hold for **5 mins**
on each side

hold for **5 mins**
on each side

hold for **5 mins**

Increasing hamstring flexibility

This sequence focuses on the connective tissues around your hamstrings for increased flexibility in your lower body. The asanas specifically target your legs, which can become overly stiff due to prolonged sitting.

REQUIRED PROPS
- 1 strap
- 1 block

OPTIONAL PROP
- 1 additional block

START	SEATED MEDITATION page 24	HUMMING BEE BREATH page 19	RECLINED BUTTERFLY page 54	RECLINING LEG STRETCH 1 (right side) page 30	RECLINING LEG STRETCH 2 (right side) page 32
	● hold for **6 mins** »	● hold for **5 mins** »	● hold for **5 mins** »	● hold for **3 mins** »	● hold for **3 mins** »

DRAGON FLYING LOW (right side) page 94	HALF MONKEY (right side) page 140	DRAGON FLYING LOW (left side) page 94
● hold for **5 mins** »	● hold for **5 mins** »	● hold for **5 mins** »

RECLINING LEG STRETCH 3 (right side) page 34	**RECLINING LEG STRETCH 1** (left side) page 30	**RECLINING LEG STRETCH 2** (left side) page 32	**RECLINING LEG STRETCH 3** (left side) page 34	**CATERPILLAR** page 48
hold for **3 mins**	hold for **3 mins**	hold for **3 mins**	hold for **3 mins**	hold for **5 mins**

HALF MONKEY (left side) page 140	**MONKEY** page 142	**SUPPORTED BRIDGE** page 98	**LYING SPINAL TWIST** page 60	**CORPSE** page 144	FINISH
hold for **5 mins**	hold for **5 mins** on each side	hold for **5 mins**	hold for **5 mins** on each side	hold for **6 mins**	

TOTAL TIME »

90
minutes

Full body sequence

This sequence will remove stiffness from most joints, leaving you feeling refreshed and reinvigorated. If you start to become distracted or disengaged, bring your awareness back to your breath and take your time going in and out of the postures.

REQUIRED PROPS
• none

OPTIONAL PROPS
• 2 blocks
• 1 strap

START

SEATED MEDITATION
page 24

hold for **4 mins**

ALTERNATE NOSTRIL BREATH
page 18

perform for **5 mins**

WRIST FLEXOR STRETCH
page 70

hold for **3 mins**
on each side

WRIST EXTENSOR STRETCH
page 72

hold for **3 mins**
on each side

HALF MONKEY
page 140

hold for **5 mins**
on each side

CHILD'S POSE
page 118

BABY DRAGON
page 90

LYING QUAD STRETCH
page 58

SPHINX
page 74

hold for **5 mins**

hold for **5 mins**
on each side

hold for **5 mins**
on each side

hold for **5 mins**

SADDLE
page 62

LYING SPINAL TWIST
page 60

LEGS UP THE WALL
page 130

CORPSE
page 144

FINISH

hold for **5 mins**

hold for **5 mins**
on each side

hold for **10 mins**

hold for **4 mins**

Side body sequence

This sequence will help to open up the sides of your body – all the way from your neck down into your ribcage, hips, and outer leg – to begin to bring balance back to your entire body when you're short on time. You can work on your spinal flexibility and capacity for deep breathing by lengthening these tighter areas. This sequence may also stimulate the liver and gallbladder meridians.

REQUIRED PROPS
• none

OPTIONAL PROP
• 1 block

START

● **SEATED MEDITATION**
page 24

hold for **3 mins**

● **NECK RELEASE**
page 42

hold for **3 mins**
on each side

● **HALF BUTTERFLY**
page 52

hold for **3 mins**
on each side

● **IT BAND STRETCH**
page 40

hold for **3 mins**
on each side

● **BANANA**
page 80

hold for **3 mins**
on each side

● **CORPSE**
page 144

hold for **3 mins**

FINISH

TOTAL TIME »

60
minutes

Increasing
hip flexibility

This sequence is a great way to improve
the range of motion in your hips while also
freeing up the lower back and inner groin.
These hip-openers can also stimulate the
liver, kidney, and gallbladder meridians,
and the root and sacral chakras.

REQUIRED PROPS
• none

OPTIONAL PROPS
• 2 blocks

START

SEATED MEDITATION page 24	**HAPPY BABY** page 102	**IT BAND STRETCH** page 40	**BUTTERFLY** page 50
hold for **5 mins**	hold for **5 mins**	hold for **5 mins** on each side	hold for **10 mins**

Improving your posture

This sequence will help lengthen your spine, improve mobility in your hips and shoulders, and strengthen your posture. The energetic focus is on your stomach, kidney, and spleen meridians, plus your sacral, solar plexus, and heart chakras.

REQUIRED PROP
• 1 block

OPTIONAL PROP
• 1 block

START

SEATED MEDITATION page 24	KNEE TO CHEST page 68	SUPPORTED BRIDGE page 98	SPHINX page 74	SEAL page 76
hold for **5 mins** ≫	hold for **5 mins** on each side ≫	hold for **5 mins** ≫	hold for **5 mins** ≫	hold for **5 mins** ≫

TOTAL TIME »

60 minutes

Prenatal sequence

This sequence accommodates a growing belly during the later stages of pregnancy, when you should be avoiding twists and postures that require you to lie on your stomach. Women in their third trimester might find the Corpse uncomfortable, so you can modify it by lying on your side or performing the seated meditation again.

REQUIRED PROPS
• none

OPTIONAL PROP
• 1 block

START

SEATED MEDITATION page 24	NECK RELEASE page 42	DANGLING page 84	SQUAT page 36	HALF BUTTERFLY page 52
hold for **5 mins**	hold for **5 mins** on each side	hold for **5 mins**	hold for **5 mins**	hold for **5 mins** on each side

BUTTERFLY
page 50

ANKLE STRETCH
page 44

SEAL
page 76

CHILD'S POSE
(do the variation)
page 118

CORPSE (on your side)
page 144
or
SEATED MEDITATION
page 24

FINISH

 hold for **5 mins**

 hold for **3 mins**
on each side

hold for **3 mins**

hold for **5 mins**

hold for **6 mins**

TOTAL TIME »

60 minutes

Chakra opener

These asanas will open up your chakras one by one, starting with the root chakra at the base of the spine and going all the way up to the crown chakra at the top of the head. Feel and visualize the rise of energy through your chakras as you hold these postures. This is a meditative sequence that includes two seated meditations for introspection and reflection.

REQUIRED PROPS
• 2 blocks or a bolster

OPTIONAL PROPS
• none

START

SEATED MEDITATION page 24	DEER page 110	WINGED DRAGON page 96	LYING SPINAL TWIST page 60	SPHINX page 74
hold for **5 mins**	hold for **5 mins** on each side	hold for **5 mins** on each side	hold for **5 mins** on each side	hold for **5 mins**

SUPPORTED FISH
page 124

CHILD'S POSE
page 118

SEATED MEDITATION
page 24

CORPSE
page 144

FINISH

hold for **5 mins**   hold for **5 mins**   hold for **5 mins**   hold for **5 mins**

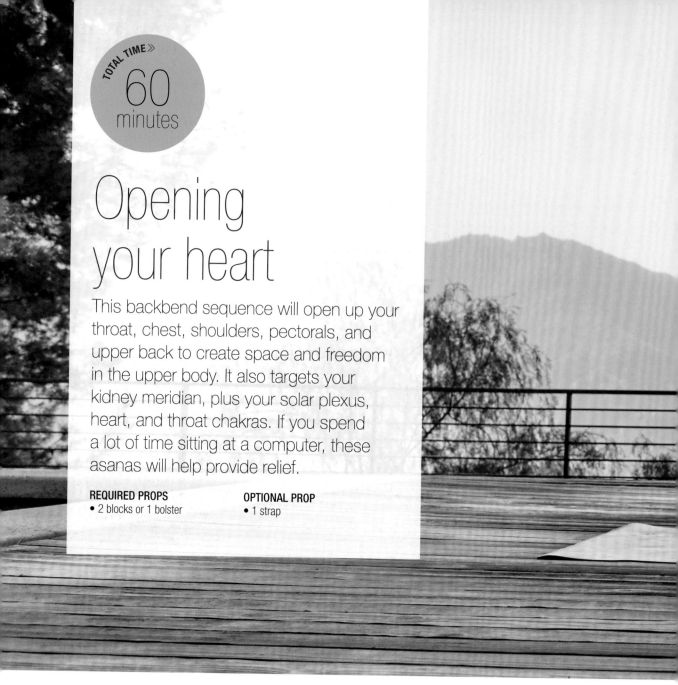

TOTAL TIME »

60
minutes

Opening
your heart

This backbend sequence will open up your throat, chest, shoulders, pectorals, and upper back to create space and freedom in the upper body. It also targets your kidney meridian, plus your solar plexus, heart, and throat chakras. If you spend a lot of time sitting at a computer, these asanas will help provide relief.

REQUIRED PROPS
• 2 blocks or 1 bolster

OPTIONAL PROP
• 1 strap

START

| SEATED MEDITATION
page 24 | MELTING HEART
page 128 | SPHINX
page 74 | SEAL
page 76 | TWISTED DRAGON
page 92 |
|---|---|---|---|---|
| hold for **6 mins** » | hold for **5 mins** » | hold for **5 mins** » | hold for **3 mins** » | hold for **5 mins**
on each side » |

SADDLE page 62	**REVERSE PRAYER ARMS** page 136	**SUPPORTED FISH** page 124	**RECLINED CHILD'S POSE** page 120	**CORPSE** page 144	FINISH
hold for **5 mins**	hold for **5 mins**	hold for **10 mins**	hold for **5 mins**	hold for **6 mins**	

Index

About the author

Kassandra Reinhardt is an Ottawa-based yoga teacher and a leading online yin yoga instructor. Her "Yoga with Kassandra" YouTube channel has served as the gateway for thousands of people across the globe to discover the life-changing benefits of a consistent yin yoga practice. Kassandra first practised yin yoga in 2008 as a way to become more flexible and to better learn to manage stress and anxiety. The effects were so profound that she knew she wanted to become a teacher and share the same tools with others. She's passionate about sharing the gifts of yin yoga with practitioners from all around the world. Practise with her today by visiting her website at www.yogawithkassandra.com.

Acknowledgments

Thanks to everyone at DK Books for making my dream of becoming a published author a reality. Working with you has been an experience that I'll never forget. I'd especially like to thank Christopher Stolle and Brook Farling for their dedication and support throughout this process. Thank you for being open to my ideas and giving me a voice.

A big thank you to our photo shoot art director Nigel Wright and photographer Christopher Malcolm for making this book the stunning work of art that it is. Along with our fantastic models – Kelly Collins, Ryan Young, Brittany Martinez, and Q Brandon – you made the photo shoot feel like an exciting collaboration with friends, no matter how long the hours were. There was never a dull moment on set, and I appreciate your dedication and attention to detail.

A heartfelt thanks goes to my family and friends, who never cease to encourage me and are always there to lend an ear when I need it. You continuously inspire me to push myself and remind me that I can do anything I set my mind to.

Finally, I want to acknowledge my partner-in-crime, Anthony, without whom none of this would've been possible. Thank you for always being at my side, cheering me on, and believing in me even when I don't believe in myself. For standing by my side during the ups and downs and loving me through it all, this is for you.

DK UK
Senior Editor: Kate Meeker
Senior Art Editor: Glenda Fisher
Angliciser: Kate Berens
Jacket Designer: Nicola Powling
Creative Technical Support: Sonia Charbonnier
Senior Pre-production Producer: Tony Phipps
Senior Producer: Stephanie McConnell
Managing Editor: Stephanie Farrow
Managing Art Editor: Christine Keilty

DK US
Publisher: Mike Sanders
Associate Publisher: Billy Fields
Senior Editor: Brook Farling
Editor: Christopher Stolle
Book Designer: Hannah Moore
Photoshoot Art Director: Nigel Wright
Photographer: Christopher Malcolm
Prepress Technician: Brian Massey
Proofreader: Laura Caddell
Indexer: Heather McNeill

First published in Great Britain in 2018 by
Dorling Kindersley Limited
80 Strand, London, WC2R 0RL

A CIP catalogue record for this book
is available from the British Library.
ISBN: 978-0-2413-0207-1

Printed and bound in China.

All images © Dorling Kindersley Limited
For further information see: www.dkimages.com

A WORLD OF IDEAS:
SEE ALL THERE IS TO KNOW

www.dk.com